ROWAN'S
Primer of EEG

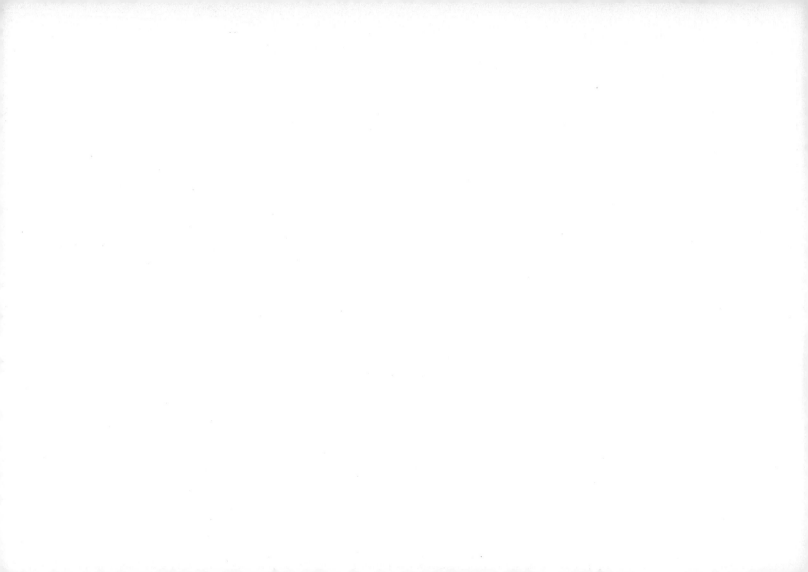

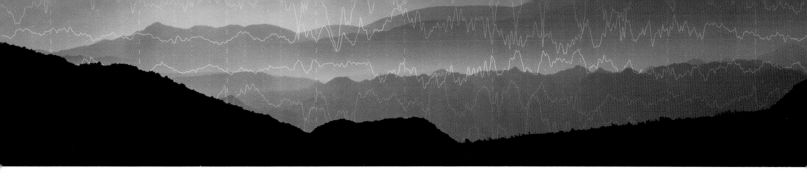

ROWAN'S

Primer of EEG

THIRD EDITION

Lara V. Marcuse, MD
Associate Professor
Department of Neurology;
Co-Director of the Mount Sinai Epilepsy Center
The Icahn School of Medicine at Mount Sinai
New York, New York

Madeline C. Fields, MD
Associate Professor
Department of Neurology;
Co-Director of the Mount Sinai Epilepsy
Center
The Icahn School of Medicine at Mount Sinai
New York, New York

Jiyeoun (Jenna) Yoo, MD
Associate Professor
Department of Neurology
The Mount Sinai Epilepsy Center
The Icahn School of Medicine at Mount Sinai
New York, New York

Foreword
Jacqueline A. French, MD
Professor
Department of Neurology
New York University Comprehensive Epilepsy Center;
Chief Scientific Officer
Epilepsy Foundation
New York, New York

ELSEVIER

For additional online content visit http://ebooks.health.elsevier.com/
Edinburgh London New York Oxford Philadelphia St Louis Sydney Toronto 2025

Elsevier
1600 John F. Kennedy Blvd.
Ste 1800
Philadelphia, PA 19103-2899

ROWAN'S PRIMER OF EEG, THIRD EDITION   ISBN: 978-0-323-75713-3

Previous editions copyrighted 2016 and 2003.

Content Strategist: Mary Hegeler
Senior Content Development Specialist: Rishi Arora
Publishing Services Manager: Shereen Jameel
Project Manager: Nandhini Thanga Alagu
Design Direction: Brian Salisbury

Printed in India

Last digit is the print number: 9 8 7 6 5 4 3 2 1

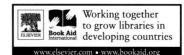

Working together
to grow libraries in
developing countries

www.elsevier.com • www.bookaid.org

*We dedicate this book to our patients (and yours as well):
past, present, and future.*

Foreword

Reading the EEG is a skill that involves both science and art. Most of us learn by apprenticeship. If you are very lucky, you learn to read with an expert sitting in the chair next to you, helping you discover the logic and the beauty of the squiggles on the page. Slowly, these squiggles that initially seem incomprehensible begin to emerge as an unfolding story. Through interpretation of the EEG (if done correctly), much is revealed about the person being tested. With time, one learns to uncover hints and clues, like a detective, that lead to a correct interpretation.

I was fortunate enough to have had A. James Rowan sitting next to me as I learned to read the EEG. Now, with his primer, updated by Marcuse, Fields and Yoo, those learning to read for the first time can benefit from a simple, easy to follow, pragmatic guide that is perfect for carrying with you to have at your side as you learn to become comfortable with the EEG. Essential information is easy to find, and the pictures and diagrams beautifully illustrate the normal and abnormal EEG. The chapter on the technical aspects of the EEG is clear, simple, and easy to follow. The illustrations of artifact have been carefully chosen, as have the normal variants and pathological epileptiform and nonepileptiform abnormalities. Each chapter provides just enough material to be helpful but not overwhelming, and there is a reference section for those seeking more in-depth information. The book will also be extremely useful to teachers of EEG, and I for one will be using the illustrations to train young encephalographers.

According to the dictionary, a primer is a book that "provides instruction in the rudiments or basic skills of a branch of knowledge." Those who master this primer will be well on their way to learning the art of EEG interpretation.

Jacqueline A. French, MD

Preface to the third edition

If I have the belief that I can do it, I shall surely acquire the capacity to do it, even if I may not have it at the beginning.

—**Mahatma Gandhi**

With this book, we seek to lay the art of reading EEGs at your feet. We have built upon the structure of the second edition. We have added two chapters: Intracranial EEG and Quantitative EEG in the ICU. Additionally, all nomenclature has been updated to the latest standards set by the International League Against Epilepsy (ILAE) and the American Clinical Neurophysiology Society (ACNS).

If you are a medical student with no intention of becoming a neurologist, we believe this primer will serve you well in understanding the EEG reports of both your outpatients and inpatients. If you are a neurologist or a neurology resident, we have included details which are useful to have at one's fingertips and easily forgotten (e.g., the meaning of subclinical rhythmic electroencephalographic discharges of adults).

As a companion to the print book, this edition can also be accessed in an electronic format, which includes a quiz for each chapter. Be warned; these questions are challenging. The answers are detailed and meant to help you integrate EEGs with clinical care and clinical decision making. Perhaps most importantly, we have created a video library of seizures. These can be watched with our annotations describing the seizure semiology and the electrographic findings, or you can choose to watch the seizures without the annotations to test your developing skill.

We will be adding to the video library with each new edition to build on your knowledge.

Learning the skill of electroencephalography may be challenging, it may be daunting, and it may not give us all the answers. However, it is a relatively inexpensive window into the workings of the brain that often provides very valuable information for diagnosis, prognosis, and management of our patients.

We hope this primer serves to increase your enthusiasm and dedication to the study of the brain, as this inquiry continues to nourish us as clinicians, teachers, and researchers.

Lara V. Marcuse, MD
Madeline C. Fields, MD
Jiyeoun (Jenna) Yoo, MD

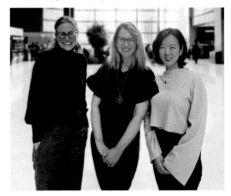

Acknowledgments

Lara Marcuse

I would like to thank my friends, family, and colleagues for all of their love and kindness. Most of all, I would like to thank my beautiful children, Cobe and Vera, who every day provide balance in my life and remind me of what's truly important. I love you to the moon and back and that is just the beginning.

Madeline Fields

To my home family, my work family and my patients, thank you from the bottom of my heart for your time, for your trust and for your love.

Jiyeoun (Jenna) Yoo

To my loving husband and our wonderful boys, Eric and Alex, who give me endless love, energy, and laughter; to my mentor, Dr. Lawrence Hirsch, who taught me all about the EEG and epilepsy with great dedication and humor; and to my current and future mentees who (I hope) find joy in this book.

We would like to thank the EEG technicians at the Mount Sinai Epilepsy Center (not program), without whom we cannot do our work. Specifically, the EEGs in this book were nearly all performed by a single EEG technician, Tsana Yu. Tsana Yu started with the Mount Sinai Epilepsy Center at its inception in 2009, trained on the job to become a skilled, meticulous technician, and has since trained numerous EEG technicians. Beyond that, her dedication to the patients is unparalleled. One patient's family decorated his hospital room with his paintings, and Tsana took video of the art with the VEEG camera with marks insisting that the epileptologist *look*. These gorgeous EEGs are a tribute to her ongoing work and a way for that work to continue to teach others.

Finally, we wish to thank the following colleagues for their contributions:

Chapter 1: James J. Young, MD, PhD, Icahn School of Medicine at Mount Sinai.

Chapter 2: Weiyi Gao, MD, Icahn School of Medicine at Mount Sinai.

Chapter 3: Maite La Vega-Talbott, MD, Mount Sinai Kravis Children's Hospital.

Chapter 4: Anuradha Singh, MD, Icahn School of Medicine at Mount Sinai.

Chapter 5: Leah J. Blank, MD, MPH, Icahn School of Medicine at Mount Sinai.

Chapter 8: Hae Young Baang, MD, Icahn School of Medicine at Mount Sinai.

Chapter 9: Kyusang S. Lee, MD, Icahn School of Medicine at Mount Sinai.

Appendix 1: Dong-Hee Kim, MD, PIH Health.

Appendix 1: Jessica Yen, MD, Specialty Care (IOM).

Appendix 2: Gabriela B. Tantillo, MD, MPH, Baylor College of Medicine.

Q&A Section: Kapil Gururangan, MD, Department of Neurology, University of California Los Angeles.

In addition, we would like to thank the wonderful neurosurgeons with whom we work, Saadi Ghatan, MD and Fedor Panov, MD.

Contents

Origin and technical aspects of the EEG 1

ORIGIN OF THE EEG

The EEG measures the electrical activity coming from the brain, but several factors influence the brain activity as measured on the scalp. Because of the insulating effect of the skull, the distance between the brain and the EEG electrode and background activity in the room, the part of the electrical signal that is from the brain is very small, measured in microvolts (μV), and may be undetectable. The activity is so small that it must be amplified by a factor of 1,000,000 to be usefully represented for human eyes. Furthermore, the amount of brain tissue that is required to generate a signal that is detectable on the scalp is relatively large. At least 6–10 cm^2 of simultaneously activated cortex is required for that activity to be measured on the scalp.

The composition of the underlying brain signal is similarly complex. Scalp EEGs measure the local field potential (LFP), or the sum of extracellular potentials from the tissues near the detecting electrode. The conventional assumption was that the primary component of the LFP is from synaptic potentials from neurons. This assumption was based on the observation that action potentials are too fast and too asynchronized to contribute largely to the LFP. However, recent data suggest that action potentials, calcium spikes, intrinsic oscillators, and neuron-glia interactions via gap junctions can all influence the LFP and hence the scalp EEG. This field continues to evolve, and many early assumptions have been found wanting. For example, it was also assumed that EEG activity

is primarily from pyramidal neurons, but recordings from humans and nonhuman primates suggest that the LFP is primarily from interneurons as opposed to pyramidal cells.

Still, at present, postsynaptic potentials (PSPs) are thought by many to be the largest source for the signal measured by EEG. The resting membrane potential (electrochemical equilibrium) is typically −70 mV (inside minus outside by convention). At the postsynaptic membrane, neurotransmitters produce a change in membrane conductance and the transmembrane potential. If the neurotransmitter has an excitatory effect on the neuron, it leads to a local reduction of the transmembrane potential (depolarization) and is called an excitatory postsynaptic potential (EPSP). Note that during an EPSP, the inside of the neuronal membrane becomes more positive, while the extracellular matrix becomes more negative. By contrast, inhibitory postsynaptic potentials (IPSPs) result in local hyperpolarization, with the transmembrane potential becoming more negative. Thus this model proposes that the LFP is composed of the sum of EPSPs and IPSPs, so the EEG primarily measures the voltage changes in the extracellular matrix associated with neurotransmitter release at the synapse.

Neuronal electrical activity generates irregular LFP signals, which are then recorded as seemingly random and ever-changing EEG waves. However, the physiological explanation of the rhythmic character of certain EEG patterns is even more complicated. The mechanism of EEG rhythmicity, although not completely understood, is likely mediated through two main processes. The first is the interaction between cortex and thalamus. The activity of thalamic pacemaker cells leads to rhythmic cortical activation. For example, the cells in the nucleus reticularis of the thalamus have the pacing properties responsible for the generation of sleep spindles. The second is based on the functional properties of neuronal networks that have an intrinsic capacity for rhythmicity. For example, synchronous activity in diffuse networks is detected during the performance of memory, perception, and attention tasks, and it is thought that this rhythmic activity is necessary for the performance of these tasks by organizing disparate brain regions into networks. Thus rhythmicity observed on EEG may be created by thalamocortical loops and the intrinsic properties of cortical networks. Both mechanisms help create recognizable EEG patterns that allow readers to differentiate normal from abnormal activity.

TECHNICAL CONSIDERATIONS

The essence of EEG is the amplification of tiny brain signals into a graphic representation that can be interpreted. Unfortunately, no technology currently exists that can fully separate cerebral from extracerebral signals like motion artifact or noise from electrical devices. As a consequence, extracerebral potentials are likewise amplified, and these are frequently many times the amplitude of electrocortical potentials. Thus unless understood and corrected for, such interference or artifacts obscure the underlying brain signals. Trained electoencephalographers seek to fully understand these artifacts in order to discern the brain signals beneath them. Later, we will discuss artifacts in detail and illustrate clearly their many guises. At this point, we will consider the technical factors that are indispensable in obtaining an interpretable record.

Electrodes

Electrodes are simply the means by which the electrocortical potentials are conducted to the amplification apparatus. Essentially, standard EEG electrodes are small, nonreactive metal discs or cups applied to the scalp with a conductive paste. Several types of metals are used, including gold, silver, tin, and platinum. Electrode contact must be firm in order to ensure low impedance (resistance to current flow), minimizing both electrode and environmental artifacts. For long-term monitoring, especially if the patient is mobile, cup electrodes are affixed with an adhesive substance and a conductive gel is inserted between the electrode and the scalp through a small hole in the electrode itself. This procedure maintains recording integrity over prolonged periods.

Other types of electrodes are available, including plastic as well as needle electrodes. In fact, some plastic electrodes are MRI compatible. Needle electrodes, which in the past were often used in ICUs, have been redeveloped and consist of a painless subdermal electrode.

Electrode placement

Electrode placement is standardized in the United States and indeed in most other nations. This allows EEGs performed in one laboratory to be interpreted in another. The general problem is to record activity from various parts of the cerebral cortex in a logical, interpretable manner. Thanks to Dr. Herbert Jasper, a renowned electroencephalographer at the Montreal Neurological Institute, we have a logical and generally accepted system of electrode placement: the 10-20 International System of Electrode Placement (Fig. 1.1). The 10-10 system (Fig. 1.2) is similar but has slightly different numbering. The 10-10 system was constructed so that if additional electrodes are to be placed on the scalp, there is a logical numbering system with which to do so.

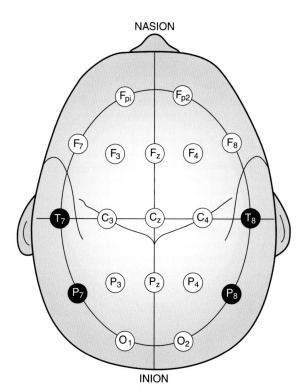

NASION

INION

FIGURE 1.1 10-20 system. A single-plane projection of the head showing all standard positions and the locations of the Rolandic and Sylvian fissures. The outer circle was drawn at the level of the nasion and inion. The inner circle represents the temporal line of electrodes. T7, T8, P7 and P8 used to be referred to as T3, T4, T5 and T6.

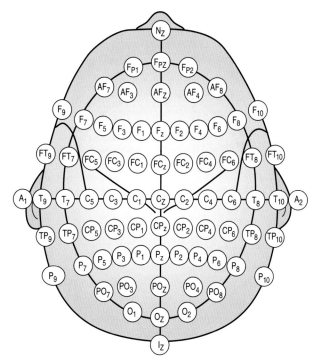

FIGURE 1.2 10-10 system. The 10-20 system has been modified to standardize a method for adding more electrodes.

Table 1.1 Standard electrode designations

Left	Right	Electrode
		Parasagittal/suprasylvian electrodes
Fp1	Fp2	Frontopolar, located on the forehead—postscripted numbers are different than other electrodes in this sagittal line (3,4)
F3	F4	Midfrontal
C3	C4	Central—roughly over the central sulcus
P3	P4	Parietal
O1	O2	Occipital-postscripted numbers are different from other electrodes in this sagittal line (3,4)
		Lateral/temporal electrodes
F7	F8	Inferior frontal/anterior temporal
T7	T8	Midtemporal—formerly T3, T4
P7	P8	Posterior temporal/parietal—formerly T5,T6
		Other electrodes
Fz, Cz, Pz		Midline electrodes: frontal, central, and parietal
A1	A2	Earlobe electrodes. Often used as reference electrodes from the contralateral side. Of note, they record ipsilateral midtemporal activity
LLC	RUC	Left lower canthus/right upper canthus (placed on the lower and upper outer corners of the eyes). These electrodes are used to detect eye movements and can help distinguish eye movements from brain activity. Sometimes designated LOC, ROC.

Both the 10-10 and 10-20 systems depend on accurate measurements of the skull, utilizing several distinctive landmarks. Measurements of the skull are taken in three planes—sagittal, coronal, and horizontal. Electrodes designated with odd numbers are on the left; those with even numbers are on the right. Standard electrode designations and placement should be memorized by every EEG student during the first day of their elective (Table 1.1).

How to measure for electrode placement
Sagittal plane. The sagittal measurement starts at the nasion (the depression at the top of the nose) over the top of the head to the inion (the prominence in the midline at the base of the occiput). With a red wax pencil, mark the point above the nasion that is 10% of the total measurement (Fpz) and the point above the inion that also is 10% of the total (Oz). These locations are used as coordinates to help identify the

other designated electrode destinations. Divide and mark the remaining 80% into four segments, each 20% of the total measurement. The first 20% point is Fz, the second Cz, and the third Pz—the midline electrodes (z = zero). The final 20% is the distance between Pz and the point 10% above the inion (Oz). Thus the total is 100% (Fig. 1.3A).

Coronal plane. The coronal plane extends from the point anterior to the tragus (the cartilaginous protrusion at the front of the external ear) to the same point on the opposite side, making sure that the tape measure traverses the Cz point on the sagittal measurement. The intersection of the halfway (50%) points of the sagittal and coronal measurements is the location of the vertex and thus the Cz electrode. The first 10%

points up from the tragus define T7 and T8, the midtemporal electrodes. The next 20% points then define C3 and C4, the central electrodes. The remaining 20% segments represent the distances from C3 to Cz and Cz to C4 (Fig. 1.3B).

Horizontal plane. The trickiest measurements are in the horizontal plane. The horizontal plane is generated with a measurement from Fpz to T7 to Oz on the left and from Fpz to T8 to Oz on the right. Fp1 and Fp2 are placed on either side of Fpz, both at a distance of 5% of the total horizontal circumference from Fpz. Similarly, O1 and O2 are placed at a 5% distance of the total horizontal circumference from Oz. The distances from Fp1 to F7 to T7 to P7 to O1 on the left and from Fp2 to F8 to T8

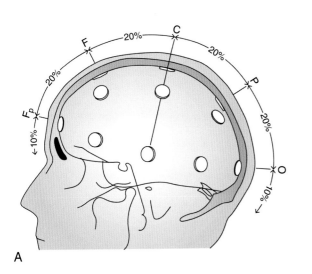

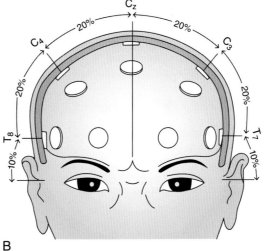

A

B

FIGURE 1.3 **Measurements in the 10-10 system in the (A) sagittal, (B) coronal, and (C) horizontal planes.** (A) Lateral view of the skull to show the method of measurement from the nasion to inion at the midline. Fp is the frontal pole position, F is the frontal line of electrodes, C is the central line, P is the parietal line, and O is the occipital line. Percentages indicate proportions of the total measurement from the nasion to the inion. The central line is 50% of this distance. (B) Frontal view of the skull showing the coronal measurements.

to P8 to O2 on the right are all 10% of the total horizontal circumference (Fig. 1.3C). Finally, F3 and F4 are defined by the halfway points between F7 and Fz on the left and F8 and Fz on the right. Similarly, P3 and P4 are defined by the halfway points between P7 and Pz on the left and P8 and Pz on the right.

In the 10-10 system, there are remaining electrode positions in the 10% intermediate lines between the existing standard coronal and sagittal lines. It is best to look at Fig. 1.2 while reading the next several sentences. Coronally, these electrode positions are named by combining the designation of the coronal lines anterior and posterior. For example, the coronal line between the parietal (P) and occipital (O) chains is designated PO. The only exception is in the first intermediate coronal line, which is named anterior frontal (AF) rather than FpF or FF. In the sagittal line, the same postscript numbers are used; for example, AF3, F3, FC3, C3, CP3, P3, and PO3. From the midline, moving laterally, the postscript begins at z followed by the numbers 1, 3, 5, 7, 9 on the left and 2, 4, 6, 8, 10 on the right. We now have the 10-10 system in which each letter appears on only one coronal line and each postscripted number on a sagittal line (*except for* Fp1/Fp2 and O1/O2). The 10-10 system locates each electrode at the intersection of a specific coronal (identified by the letter) and sagittal (identified by the number) line.

An observation. The F7 and F8 electrodes are probably placed too high for optimal definition of anterior temporal activity. Likewise, the P7 and P8 electrodes are probably too high for good definition of posterior temporal activity. Thus it is possible to logically place additional electrodes (F9/F10, T9/T10, and P9/P10), which are placed 10% inferior to the standard (F7/8, T7/8, P7/8, respectively) electrodes. In some laboratories, these additional electrodes are routinely used.

While the 10-10 system may sound slightly complicated, it is quite easily carried out in practice. Nonetheless, there is nothing like actually

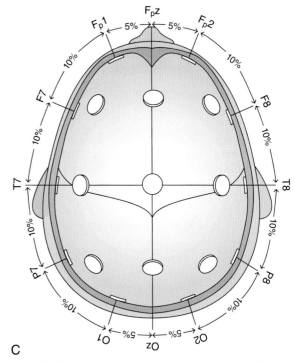

C

FIGURE 1.3, cont'd (C) Superior view with cross section of the skull through the temporal line of electrodes.

measuring and placing the electrodes under the guidance of an experienced EEG technician and performing at least two to three supervised EEGs during the EEG rotation. Fellows should do more until they are confident in their ability to measure accurately and apply electrodes properly.

Potential fields

Before discussing how we display the electrical information recorded by the electrodes, the reader should understand the concept of the potential field. The summation of IPSPs and EPSPs in a neuronal net creates electrical currents that flow in and around the cells. The flow of current creates a field that spreads out from the origin of an electrical event (such as a spike or slow wave), much the same as the concentric rings created on a glassy pond when one tosses a pebble onto its surface. Potential fields may be quite restricted or very widespread. The field's effect diminishes as the distance from the source increases. This means that events producing maximal voltage on a particular electrode will affect adjacent electrodes as well but to a lesser extent as the potential wanes from the point of origin (Fig. 1.4).

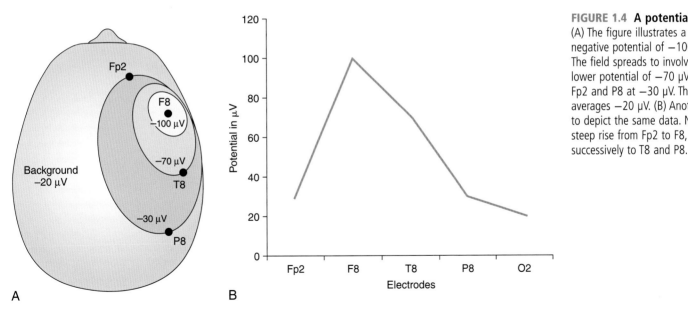

A   B

FIGURE 1.4 A potential field.
(A) The figure illustrates a maximum negative potential of −100 μV at F8. The field spreads to involve T8 at a lower potential of −70 μV and then to Fp2 and P8 at −30 μV. The background averages −20 μV. (B) Another way to depict the same data. Note the steep rise from Fp2 to F8, declining successively to T8 and P8.

Amplification

The input from an active electrode is conducted to the amplifier and compared with a reference electrode; thus the output consists of the potential difference between the active electrode and the reference. Modern amplifiers are digital, meaning that this potential difference is converted to a digital signal. As noted, electrocortical potentials, as well as other environmental potentials affecting the electrode (e.g., 60 Hz noise), are included in the output, so amplifiers are designed to remove or minimize environmental potentials. For older analog amplifiers, this was done using different reference schemes (called montages) to address noise and artifacts with recording. An example is a process called differential amplification. In differential amplification, signals from two active leads are conducted to the amplifier, thus measuring the potential difference between the two (Fig. 1.5). Any signal that affects both inputs identically (say 60 Hz) will result in no potential difference and thus will not be displayed or be much reduced. This phenomenon is termed in-phase cancellation. Digital amplifiers use very similar approaches, but these are implemented on the digital signal after it has been recorded. The process is similar; it is just implemented by the software rather than the hardware.

We are now in a position to consider methods of recording electrocortical potentials so that we can make sense of them. Recalling that amplifiers record potential difference between two incoming signals, we can record the potential difference between two electrodes on the scalp (bipolar recording). On the other hand, we can record the potential difference between a scalp electrode and another point (the reference) that ideally is unaffected by cerebral potentials or other interference (referential recording). Unfortunately, it is virtually impossible to achieve this ideal, but certain references (e.g., the ears) are quite serviceable. These

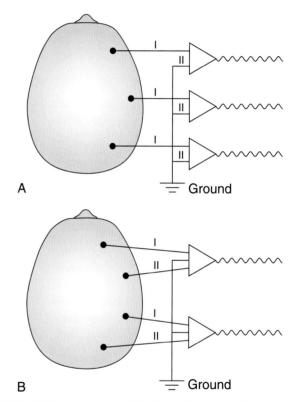

FIGURE 1.5 (A) Simple analog amplifier. Input from each active electrode is compared with that of the reference. (B) Differential amplifier. Here, potential difference is measured between two active electrodes.

two types of recordings, along with their advantages and disadvantages, are discussed below.

Bipolar recording

Bipolar recordings measure the potential differences between successive electrodes (known as a chain or line). The voltage at one electrode is compared with the voltage affecting adjacent electrodes. Each amplifier has two inputs, I and II. By convention, the rules for understanding the display are:

> If input I becomes negative with respect to input II, there is an upward deflection.
> If input II becomes negative with respect to input I, there is a downward deflection.

Note that contrary to the Cartesian coordinate system, the convention in neurophysiology is that an upward deflection is negative and a downward deflection is positive.

In the simplest example, consider a spike with a very limited potential field involving only T8 (Fig. 1.6). The electrode pairs (or derivations) in this case are F8–T8 and T8–P8. F8–T8 is channel 1 and T8–P8 is channel 2. In channel 1, T8 is in input II, and in channel 2, T8 is in input I. The voltage at T8 (-100 µV) is compared with the background activity at F8 and P8 (-20 µV). Therefore, in this example:

Channel 1: F8–T8 = -20 µV $-$ (-100 µV) = 80 µV (downward deflection)

Channel 2: T8–P8 = (-100 µV) $-$ (-20 µV) = -80 µV (upward deflection)

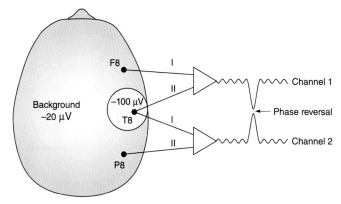

FIGURE 1.6 Principle of bipolar localization. The figure depicts a spike discharge of -100 µV at T8. The potential is conducted to input II in the first amplifier and to input I in the second amplifier. Other electrodes are not affected by the event. The result is known as a phase reversal.

In this case, the adjacent channels containing the T8 electrode record the same potential but in opposite directions. This creates the phase reversal. Most spike discharges at the surface are negative in sign, and negative phase reversals resemble two sharp points touching or nearly touching (remember, if you tried to put your finger through a *negative* phase reverse, it might get pricked and be a *negative* experience). Channels 1 and 2 are displaying the same potential but with opposite deflections. Again, this is phase reversal. Phase reversal is a localization principle of bipolar recording because it helps identify where a potential is maximal.

Let us now analyze the display when a spike at F8 has a wider potential field that also affects Fp2 and T8 (Fig. 1.7A). In channel 1, the

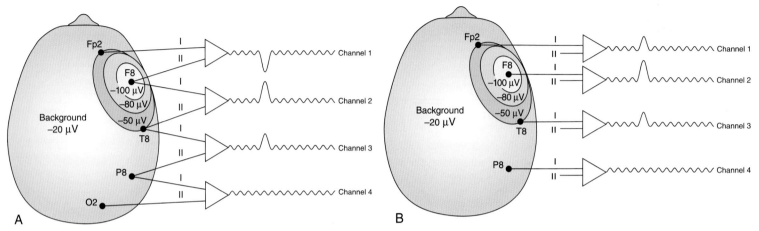

FIGURE 1.7 (A) Phase reversal in longitudinal bipolar montage. Here, a spike of $-100\ \mu V$ at F8 spreads to involve Fp2 and T8, each at $-50\ \mu V$. The potential difference between F8 and the other two electrodes is 50 μV. The display demonstrates a phase reversal at F8 (channels 1 and 2), with lower amplitude representation of the spike in channel 3 (the potential difference between T8 and P8 is $-30\ \mu V$). (B) Referential montage. The same spike displayed in a referential montage. In a referential montage, each electrode is compared to a reference electrode. The potential at the active electrode is conducted to input I of each amplifier. The reference electrode is conducted to input II. The amplitude of the displayed spike is proportional to the voltage at each active electrode.

voltage at Fp2 ($-50\ \mu V$) is compared with the voltage at F8 ($-100\ \mu V$). In channel 2, the voltage at F8 ($-100\ \mu V$) is compared with the voltage at T8 ($-50\ \mu V$). In channel 3, the voltage at T8 ($-50\ \mu V$) is compared to the voltage P8, which is unaffected by the spike at F8 but is recording the background activity ($-20\ \mu V$). In channel 4, the voltage at P8 is compared with O2, both unaffected by the F8 spike. Thus there is no potential difference and no deflection.

Channel 1: Fp2–F8 $= (-50\ \mu V) - (-100\ \mu V) = 50\ \mu V$ (downward deflection)

Channel 2: F8–T8 $= (-100\ \mu V) - (-50\ \mu V) = -50\ \mu V$ (upward deflection)

Channel 3: T8–P8 $= (-50\ \mu V) - (-20\ \mu V) = -30\ \mu V$ (a smaller upward deflection)

Channel 4: P8–O2 $= (-20\ \mu V) - (-20\ \mu V) = 0\ \mu V$ (no deflection)

Other channels (e.g., F4–C4 and C4–P4) may be affected by the declining potential field generated at F8. Thus phase reversals at lower amplitude would be recorded at these sites. Note that these considerations apply to any potential at any point on the scalp.

Referential recording

In referential recording, the potential differences are not calculated relative to neighboring electrodes. Rather, they are calculated relative to a selected "reference" electrode. For digital amplifiers, this is not necessarily the hardware reference. It is simply an electrode that is selected for every other electrode to use as a comparison. It is the same as if signals from each of the scalp electrodes are conducted to input I of the associated amplifier, while signals from the reference are conducted to input II. Thus in referential recording, we record the potential difference between a particular scalp electrode and a referential electrode. Reference montages produce a higher amplitude EEG recording because of the longer interelectrode distances. Theoretically, the reference can be located anywhere, but there are practical considerations. A reference placed at any distant point will be contaminated with ambient electrical noise, 2 Hz artifact (50 Hz in Europe). A reference placed on, say, the shoulder or chest would also pick up high-voltage EKG artifact. Interference from an EKG would render the EEG unreadable. The ears are relatively free from both these artifacts, although it must be said that EKG is sometimes a contaminant at the ear electrodes. Moreover, due to the proximity of the ears to the midtemporal lobes, the ears do pick up cerebral activity.

Now, utilizing the ears as a contralateral reference, let us compare the voltage of an event occurring at F8 with that at a contralateral ear reference, A1 (Fig. 1.7B). In this example, we will assume that A1 is recording the same as the background at −20 µV. Here we have a spike discharge with an amplitude of −100 µV at F8. The potential field of the spike spreads to Fp2 and T8 with an amplitude of −50 µV. Beyond these points, there is no representation of the field associated with the spike.

Channel 1: Fp2–A1 = (−50 µV) − (−20 µV) = −30 µV (small upward deflection)

Channel 2: F8–A1 = (−100 µV) − (−20 µV) = −80 µV (big upward deflection)

Channel 3: T8–A1 = (−50 µV) − (−20 µV) = −30 µV (small upward deflection)

Channel 4: P8–A1 = (−20 µV) − (−20 µV) = 0 µV (no deflection)

In referential recording, the localization principle is amplitude rather than phase reversal. That is, the electrode recording the greatest amplitude of the wave in question, in this case a spike at F8, defines the focus.

References other than the ears are also in common use. One is the vertex (Cz), often used in a referential montage to complement the ear reference. The astute reader will recognize that the vertex resides near an area of significant cerebral activity. Thus the background of the EEG recorded by the vertex electrode will be input II of all channels. As long as this is recognized, one is able to determine the location of a waveform that stands out from the background (e.g., a spike or delta wave).

A note on ear and vertex referential recording: a recorded event (spike, slow wave) is best represented when the reference is distant from the exploring electrode. Considering the ipsilateral ear reference (A1 or A2), the ear is close to the midtemporal electrodes T7 or T8. When examining a spike at T7, the ipsilateral ear reference (A1) is not an appropriate choice, as the potentials at T7 and A1 are very similar. A vertex reference or a contralateral ear reference (A2) is more appropriate for the examination of that T7 spike. Similarly, a spike that is maximal at C3 will be ill served by placing it in a reference montage using the Cz electrode,

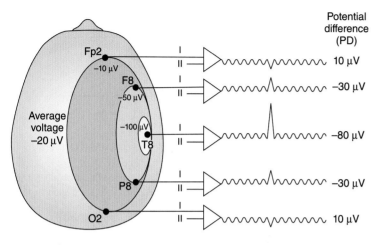

Potential difference (PD)

10 µV

−30 µV

−80 µV

−30 µV

10 µV

FIGURE 1.8 The common average reference. Recording of a spike discharge at T8 of −100 µV. The reference (going into input II at each channel) is the common average voltage, which in this case is −20 µV. In channels 2, 3, and 4, the amplitude is proportional to the recorded voltage at each electrode. The downward deflection in channels 1 and 5 is due to the fact that Fp2 and O2 are relatively electropositive (−10 µV) compared with the average voltage (−20 µV).

as the reference and the active electrode are too close together. For a C3 spike, either ear electrode would be an appropriate reference. The reference chosen for a particular spike should be as distant as possible from that spike.

Another widely used reference is the common average reference. In this scheme, the voltage of an event occurring under a particular electrode (input I) is compared with the average voltage recorded by all the electrodes on the scalp (input II). This creates a situation in which a focal spike discharge, maximal at T8, will result in an upward deflection at T8, as T8 will be more electronegative than the average reference. Neighboring electrodes involved in the field, for example at F8, will have upward deflections as well, but these will be lower in amplitude. Note that the upward deflections thus recorded define the potential field of the event. Electrodes not involved in the negative spike discharge at T8 will be relatively electropositive compared with the average reference and thus

will have a downward deflection (Fig. 1.8). Common average referencing is helpful at removing noise that is correlated between all electrodes such as environmental noise. Because this noise is present in all the averaged electrodes, it can be subtracted out and reveal the electrocerebral signal.

We now present the paradox of bipolar recording and stress how important it is to use the various montages in a complementarily fashion. The paradox is a result of the previously mentioned in-phase cancellation—that is, potentials that are equal in the two inputs of an amplifier are isoelectric in the display. In other words, there is no potential difference! The unwary, when examining channels 2 and 3 of Fig. 1.9A, might conclude that little if anything is occurring at F8, T8, and P8. On the other hand, when one looks at the same situation with a referential recording, it becomes clear that the maximum abnormality underlies those very electrodes (Fig. 1.9B). This means that it is important to review potential differences through multiple montages.

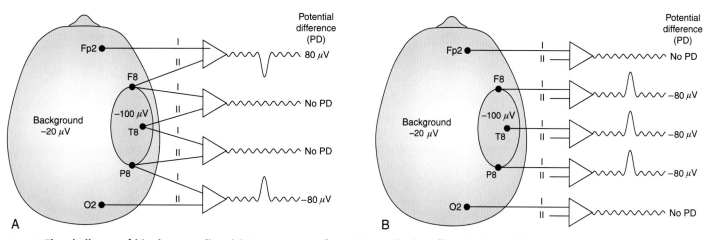

FIGURE 1.9 The challenge of bipolar recording. (A) Representation of a −100 µV spike that affects F8, T8, and P8 equally. Because there is no potential difference between F8–T8 and T8–P8, the spike is not recorded in channels 2 and 3 and gives the impression that there is no abnormality at T8. (B) Same discharge in referential recording. Note equal deflection in channels 2, 3, and 4. The true picture is thus displayed.

Montage selection

Montage refers to the pattern of systematic linkage of the scalp electrodes designed to obtain a logical display of the electrical activity. Unlike the 10-10 system of electrode placement described earlier, there is no international standard of montages to be used in EEG laboratories. Certain montages, however, are in widespread use. In bipolar recording the longitudinal arrangement is perhaps the most popular (known as the "double banana," and by some as the Queen Square montage) (Fig. 1.10A). Note: Arrows are often used in North America for convenience: the tail of the arrow indicates input I and the point of the arrow input II.

Adjacent electrodes are connected from front to back, including the temporal (lateral) chain and the parasagittal (suprasylvian) chain. The EEG is displayed in various ways. In this example, the four channels of the temporal chain on one side are followed by the temporal channels on the opposite side. Similarly, the four channels of the parasagittal chain also alternate. In North America, the left side is written out first, followed by the right. In Europe, the opposite is the case. Some laboratories write out the eight channels of left-sided electrodes, followed by the right-sided electrodes. Still others prefer alternating homologous channels, for example, Fp1 → F7; Fp2 → F8, and so on. Overall, the latter tends to be

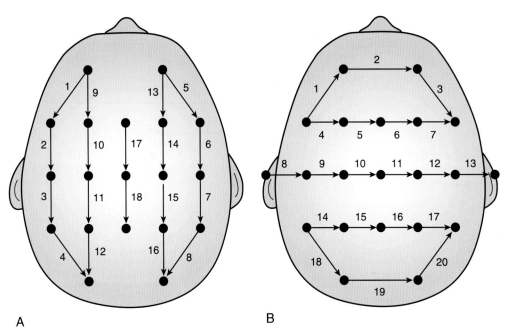

A

B

FIGURE 1.10 (A) A typical longitudinal bipolar montage. The numbers refer to channels, reflecting voltage difference between two electrodes. Both temporal and suprasylvian chains alternate from left to right. The *arrows* represent the inputs to each amplifier. The *tail* is in input I and the *arrow* is in input II. (B) A transverse bipolar montage. The chains run from left to right, beginning anteriorly and proceeding posteriorly. Note that the midline electrodes are incorporated into the second, third, and fourth chains, thus allowing good representation of midline events.

a bit more confusing—but electroencephalographers experienced with a particular electrode arrangement have no difficulty.

A second popular arrangement is the transverse bipolar montage. This links adjacent electrodes in transverse chains, starting anteriorly and progressing posteriorly. Each chain starts with the left side and progresses to the right (i.e., F7 → F3 → Fz → F4 → F8). The transverse montage is particularly well suited to record abnormalities occurring at or near the

vertex (e.g., midline spikes) (Fig. 1.10B). One additional bipolar montage comes to mind: the circumferential montage. As the name implies, the circumferential montage encircles the head and is particularly useful for examining spikes and sharp waves, which occur at the end of the longitudinal bipolar chain: Fp1, Fp2, O1, or O2 (Figs. 1.10C and 1.11).

With respect to referential recording, the recording is usually displayed in both anterior-posterior and transverse arrangements, reprising

In the era of digital EEG, specific montage selection by the technologist is not as critical as it was in the analog days. All recording is actually done referentially. The software allows the display of recorded potentials in any desired montage. Thus the technician and reader can now easily switch from one montage to another to examine the characteristics of a particular phenomenon. A low-amplitude temporal spike during bipolar recording can rapidly be inspected on a referential montage with a click of the computer mouse.

In summary, the technologist may record an EEG in a set sequence of montages, but the reviewing electroencephalographer can review the EEG in any montage desired. Furthermore, a given page or discharge can be examined in a variety of montages to help understand its meaning. Much as we would circle a complex sculpture in a museum, we circle an EEG wave by using different montages. Remember, the idea is to maximize the opportunity to display an abnormality for optimal recognition.

SOFTWARE OVERVIEW

The EEG display can be manipulated at will and made to demonstrate a severe abnormality or to show a normal pattern. This manipulation refers to the manner of digital representation to alter sensitivity, filtration, and time base. While there are a wide variety of settings that can change this digital representation, for many years, nearly all laboratories in North America and indeed many laboratories throughout the world have used similar electronic settings for routine work. This is so that EEGs obtained in one laboratory are easily interpretable at another. The following is a brief discussion of the most important recording parameters.

Calibration and impedance

Calibration is a way to accurately measure the size of EEG potentials by administrating a standard signal through each amplifier. Once this

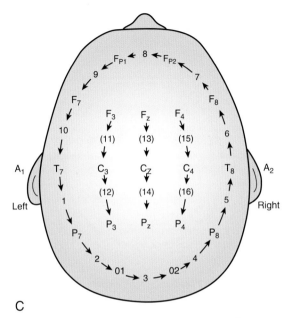

C

FIGURE 1.10, cont'd (C) Circumferential bipolar montage. This montage allows for the visualization of phase reversal at the occipital and frontopolar electrodes, which are at the end of the chain in the typical longitudinal bipolar montage.

commonly used bipolar montages. A variety of other montages are employed at the discretion of the individual electroencephalographer. The idea, in short, is to highlight certain areas of interest in the best possible way. If the student is familiar with the 10-10 system and is apprised of the montage, they should have no difficulty in interpreting the record.

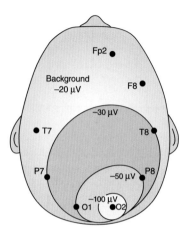

FIGURE 1.11 **Occipital spike.** Spike discharges at the "end of chain (Fp1, Fp2, O1, O2)" can be easy to miss in the standard longitudinal bipolar montage. Here, a right occipital (O2) spike discharge is displayed at −100 µV. (A) In a standard longitudinal bipolar montage, the deflection is always downward. (B) The discharge can be confirmed by placing it in a circumferential bipolar montage. Phase reversal at O2 confirms the spike maximum at this location.

is performed, the voltage of an EEG potential is compared against this known voltage. Calibration is currently built into the software of most digital EEG systems and is performed automatically. Additionally, an impedance check should appear at the start of every recording. The impedance check is a way of establishing the integrity of each electrode. Impedances should not exceed 5 kohm.

Display

In most North American and many European laboratories, the standard display time base is 30 mm/s, with 10 seconds of EEG per display. There is nothing magical about the number—in fact, some laboratories (particularly in Europe) prefer a time base of 15 mm/s. The appearance of the EEG is considerably altered in the latter case (i.e., the alpha rhythm at 30 mm/s looks like rhythmic beta activity at 15 mm/s). The important point is that the reader knows which time base is selected. It should be said that there are instances when a shorter time base is quite useful (e.g., in the identification of periodicity, or even rhythmicity of a particular phenomenon [e.g., in ICUs or for neonatal EEGs]). Likewise, increasing the time base to, say, 60 mm/s may allow one to analyze more accurately the location of maximal activity at seizure onset.

Longitudinal bipolar montage	Potential difference (PD)	Circumferential posterior halo	Potential difference (PD)
Fp2-F8	No PD	T8-P8	20 µV
F8-T8	10 µV	P8-O2	50 µV
T8-P8	20 µV	O2-O1	−50 µV
P8-O2	50 µV	O1-P7	−20 µV

A   B

Sensitivity

The sensitivity of each channel refers to the amplitude of the display produced by the received signal. The measurement is expressed in voltage per deflection. Standard sensitivity is 7 µV/mm.

Sensitivity may be altered for a particular channel, depending on the specific need. For example, the sensitivity of a channel recording the EKG would have to be decreased due to the much higher voltage of this signal (measured in millivolts). In general, the sensitivity of all channels recording the EEG may be changed simultaneously by a stepped gain control. For example, one might wish to increase sensitivity in situations where the general voltage of the EEG is low. Similarly, some EEG phenomena reach very high voltages (e.g., generalized spike-wave discharges), requiring a decrease in sensitivity (15 µV/mm) in order to properly analyze the waveforms. Please note that raising the gain from, for example, 7 to 15 µV is the same thing as lowering the sensitivity, and the EEG will appear lower in amplitude.

High-frequency filters (HFFs) or low-pass filters

Digital filters are frequently applied to attenuate undesirable high frequencies (e.g., muscle action potentials) and pass low frequencies (Fig. 1.12A). In an HFF analog circuit, the input signal is placed across the combination of a resistor and a capacitor in series and the output signal is measured across the capacitor alone (Fig. 1.12A). At high frequencies, the impedance of any capacitor is low. Measuring output across the capacitor with a high frequency will be essentially zero, as the voltage does not change, so the potential difference is zero. Digital filters apply similar operations to the recorded EEG signal.

The standard high frequency setting is 70 Hz. Other standard settings are 35 Hz and 15 Hz, the latter severely attenuating a broad range of high frequencies. As a practical matter, viewing at an HFF setting of 15 Hz should not be employed save in rare and unusual circumstances. An unwanted consequence would be a marked attenuation of spike potentials. Rarely, the

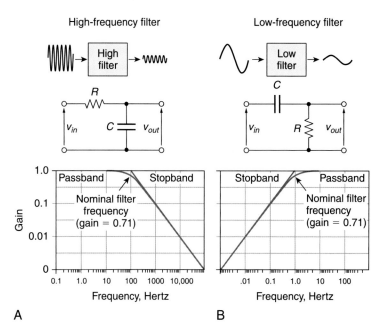

FIGURE 1.12 (A) High-frequency filter. In a high-frequency filter, the output voltage for high frequencies is lower than the input voltage for high frequencies. In the log-log graph, frequencies below the cutoff are unchanged, while frequencies above the cutoff are attenuated. (B) Low-frequency filter. In a low frequency filter, the output voltage for low frequencies is lower than the input voltage for low frequencies. In the log-log graph frequencies above the cutoffs are unchanged, while frequencies below the cutoff are attenuated. (Modified with permission from Schomer, D.L., Lopes da Silva, F.H. (Eds.), 2010. Niedermeyer's Electroencephalography. Lippincott Williams & Wilkins/Wolters Kluwer Health, Philadelphia, PA.)

seizure onset is obscured by muscle artifact, and lowering the HFF to 15 Hz can be useful in lateralizing a seizure (Fig. 1.13). More often, lowering the HFF will simply create rhythms that look "clean" but are simply aliased higher frequency activity with little underlying meaning (Fig. 1.14).

Low-frequency filters (LFFs) or high-pass filters

In an LFF, there is marked attenuation of slow potentials below the cutoff frequency (such as those caused by sweat artifact, respirations, and tongue movement), with little effect on rapid potentials such as spikes or muscle artifacts. In an LFF analog circuit, the input signal is placed across the combination of a capacitor and a resistor in series and the output signal is measured across the resistor alone (Fig. 1.12B). The impedance of any capacitor is very high at low frequencies. In this circuit arrangement, low-frequency input signals are essentially blocked. At higher frequencies, the impedance at the capacitor is low and the signal is measured across the resistor essentially unchanged from the input. Digital filters apply similar operations to the recorded EEG signal. The LFF is typically set at 1 Hz. If a recording has excessive sweat artifact, raising the LFF to 5 Hz can make the recording easier to read (Fig. 1.15).

Notch filter

In addition, a notch filter is usually employed. Alternating current electrical activity from nearby devices commonly contaminates the recorded EEG signal. In the United States, AC is at 60 Hz, whereas in Europe, it is at 50 Hz. Digital filters are applied to all the signals to reduce or mask the presence of this artifact.

NOTES ON RECORDING THE EEG

Many special problems confront technologists in their efforts to obtain an EEG that can be interpreted successfully by the electroencephalographer.

We emphasize that the electroencephalographer is totally dependent on the quality of the recording—that is, regardless of the expertise of the reader, they are unable to use that expertise in the face of technically inadequate tracing. The ability to properly place electrodes in conformity with the 10-10 International System (including, importantly, accurate measurements of electrode location) is critical if one is to compare electrical activity between the two hemispheres with accuracy. If epilepsy is suspected, the technologist should attempt to record drowsiness and sleep if possible. Moreover, because focal epileptiform activity can be activated by the interface between wakefulness and drowsiness, the technologist should gently alert the drowsy patient on several occasions to provoke spikes. Similarly, if a patient is sleeping at the onset of the test, they should be aroused after some minutes of recording. This ensures that a relative waking record is obtained. Unfortunately, sleep may obscure background abnormalities that are only evident when the patient is awake—a circumstance sometimes encountered in patients with dementia.

Artifacts

Recognition of artifacts is one of the vexing but also satisfying aspects of EEG interpretation. As a beginner, you may find the differentiation of artifacts from physiological phenomena quite difficult. A distinguishing characteristic of the experienced electroencephalographer is the ability reliably to recognize artifacts. For the most part, the reader will soon master artifact recognition, particularly after understanding their characteristics and referring to this mini-atlas, and should not be too daunted by the seeming impossibility of this task!

Artifacts come in many different forms and have diverse causes. The major underlying problem is the enormous amplification required to record brain waves. As a result, amplified noncerebral potentials—for example, vigorous movements by the patient that produce random excursions of the electrode leads—may render the EEG uninterpretable. Specific artifacts are detailed in Figs. 1.16–1.33.

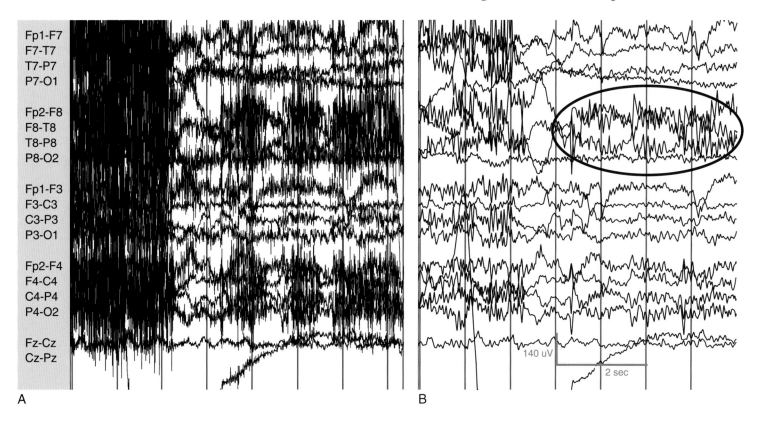

Fp1-F7
F7-T7
T7-P7
P7-O1

Fp2-F8
F8-T8
T8-P8
P8-O2

Fp1-F3
F3-C3
C3-P3
P3-O1

Fp2-F4
F4-C4
C4-P4
P4-O2

Fz-Cz
Cz-Pz

140 uV

2 sec

A

B

FIGURE 1.13 Seizure onset and the high-frequency filter (HFF). The patient has pressed the event button for her aura of fear and is sitting upright, clenching her jaw. (A) With the HFF at 70 Hz, the EEG is obscured by muscle artifact. (B) With the HFF set at 15 Hz, the first 2 seconds of EEG show muscle artifact aliased through the 15 Hz HFF filter. Then *(oval)*, rhythmic right temporal alpha can be discerned underlying the muscle artifact. This patient went on to have a right temporal lesion removed and is seizure free.

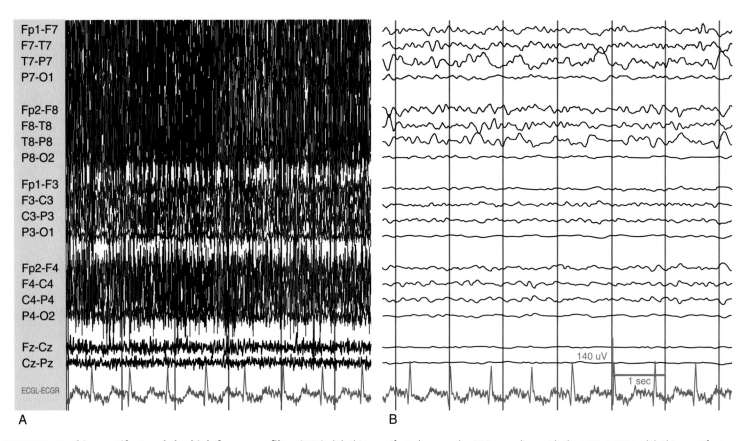

FIGURE 1.14 Shiver artifact and the high-frequency filter (HFF). (A) Shiver artifact obscures the EEG recording with the HFF at 70 Hz. (B) Shiver artifact with the HFF at 5 Hz creates the illusion of more cerebral-looking waves, but this is simply aliased shiver artifact and not brain rhythms.

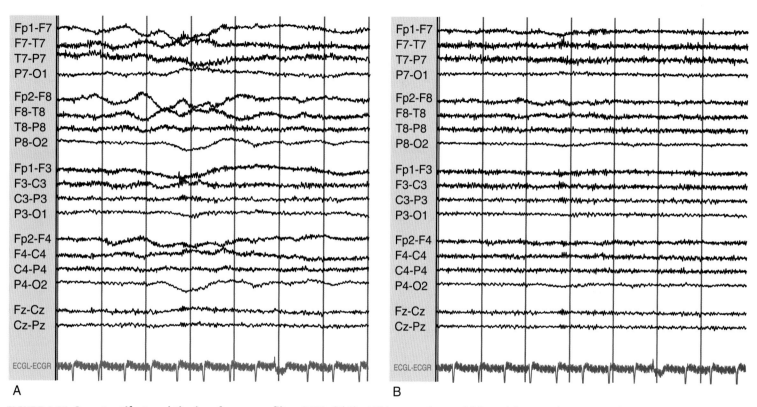

FIGURE 1.15 Sweat artifact and the low-frequency filter (LFF). (A) The LFF is set at the usual 1 Hz and the excessive sweat artifact creates visual chaos. (B) The LFF has been changed to 5 Hz, which nearly eliminates the sweat artifact without, in this case, changing the underlying cerebral rhythms.

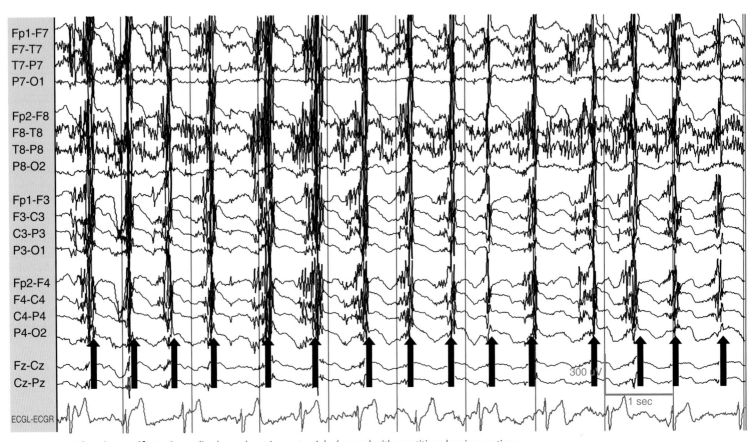

FIGURE 1.16 **Chewing artifact.** Generalized muscle action potentials *(arrows)* with repetitive chewing motions.

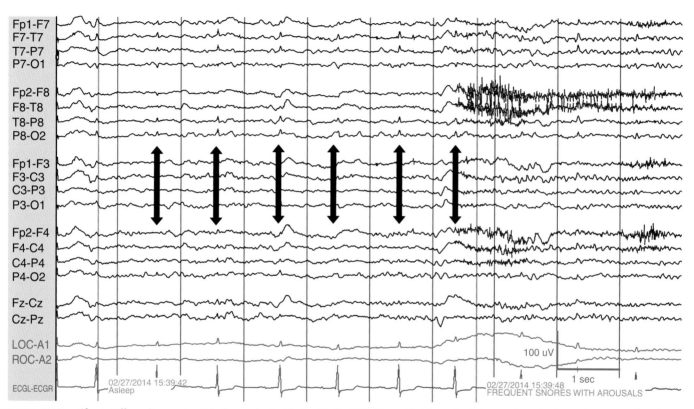

FIGURE 1.17 EKG artifact. Diffuse sharp potentials *(arrows)* coincident with the EKG. The artifact is particularly prominent in channels connected to the ears. It also may be diffuse. If there is no EKG monitor and if the patient has atrial fibrillation or frequent premature contractions, the artifact may be confounding, be inconsistent, and masquerade as spike discharges. Look for phase relationships that do not comport with those of true spikes. EKG artifact is particularly prominent in the obese and those with hypertension.

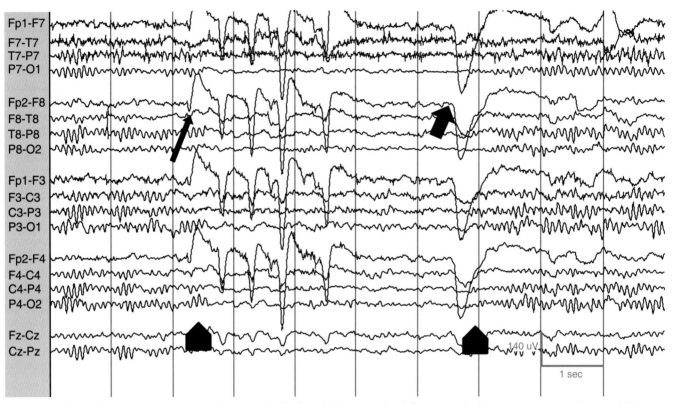

FIGURE 1.18 Eye blink artifact. High-voltage potentials, maximal in the frontal derivations. The deflection results from the cornea-retinal potential (the cornea is electropositive with respect to the retina, measured in millivolts), along with a minor contribution of the electroretinogram (ERG). During an eyeblink, the globes turn slightly upward (Bell's phenomenon). Thus the frontopolar electrodes become momentarily positive (to understand deflections, recall the rule for bipolar recording). Figure shows eye opening *(thin arrow)*, eye closure *(thick arrow)*, and disappearance and reappearance of posterior dominant rhythm (PDR) *(arrowheads)*.

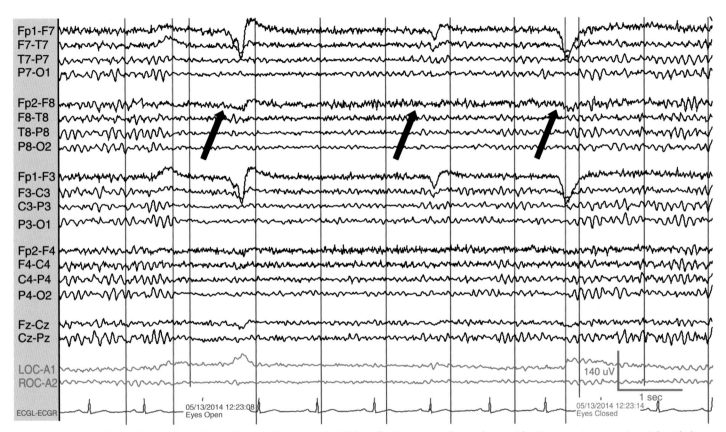

FIGURE 1.19 Prosthetic eye. In a patient with a right prosthetic eye, the blink artifact is expressed on only one side. *Arrows* point to missing right-sided eye blink artifact. One will also see limited eye blink potentials in those with a third nerve palsy.

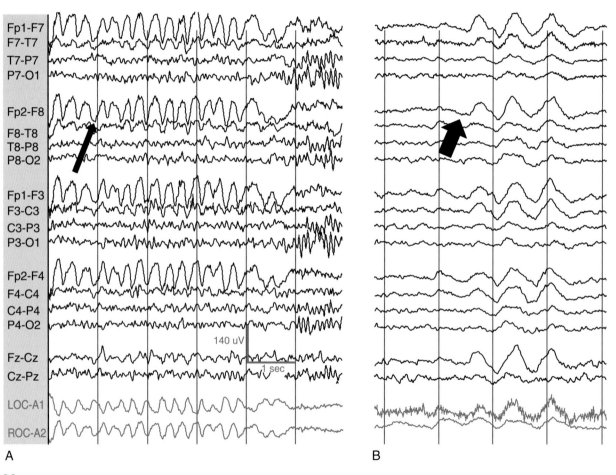

A

B

FIGURE 1.20 Eyelid flutter. In (A), eyelid flutter produces a rhythmic bifrontal frequency, here at 3–4 Hz *(thin arrow)*. Eye leads are out of phase, as left ocular (LOC) is positioned on the left lower canthus and right ocular (ROC) is positioned on the right upper canthus. (B) Shows frontally predominant, generalized rhythmic delta activity GRDA *(thick arrow)*. Eye leads show synchronous (in phase) delta, as both eye electrodes are anterior to the frontal lobe and recording very similar activity.

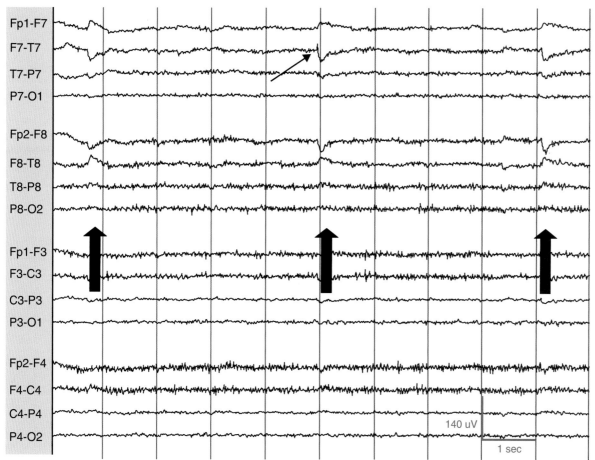

FIGURE 1.21 Lateral eye movement artifact (reading), recognizable in the frontotemporal derivations as sharply contoured potentials that are out of phase. This figure shows three left saccades *(thick arrows)*. When the eyes saccade to the left, the globe on the left approaches the left anterior temporal electrode (F7), while the right globe turns away from the right anterior temporal electrode (F8). A positive potential is therefore recorded at F7 and a negative potential at F8. (Remember, the cornea is positive with respect to the retina.) Thus in bipolar recording, the resultant waveforms deviate away from each other in the two channels connected to F7, while the opposite is the case with the channels connected to F8. Note also that very rapid spike potentials may occur during lateral eye movements with potential maxima at the F7/F8 electrodes. These result from movements of the lateral rectus muscles and are known as lateral rectus spikes *(thin arrow)*.

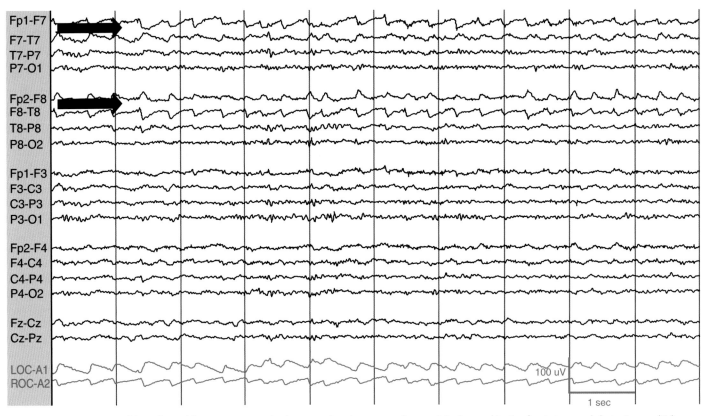

FIGURE 1.22 Nystagmus. In this patient with nystagmus, again there are sharply contoured potentials *(arrows)* in the frontotemporal derivations, which are out of phase. There is a rapid rise on the right side followed by a gradual fall, which is the corrective movement. The steeper positive phase reversal, seen here on the right, indicates the direction of the fast component of the nystagmus.

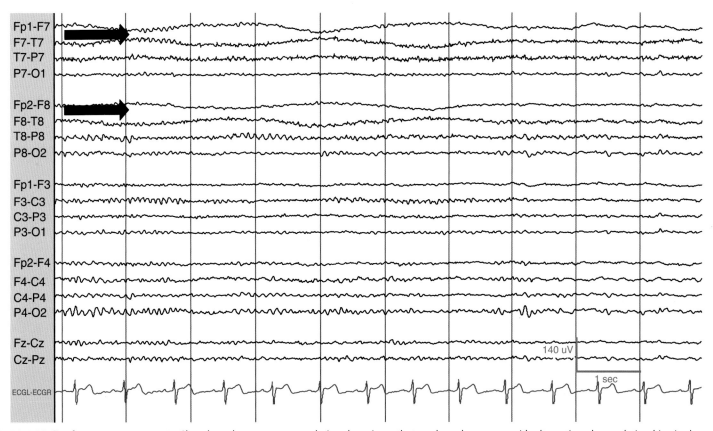

FIGURE 1.23 Roving eye movements. Slow, lateral eye movements during drowsiness that produce slow waves with alternating phase relationships in the frontotemporal derivations.

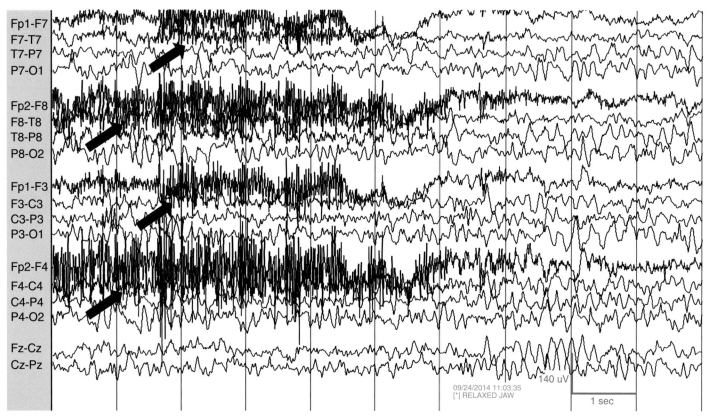

FIGURE 1.24 Muscle artifact. Muscle artifact *(arrows)* maximal in the frontal and temporal regions due to electrode placement over the frontalis and temporalis muscles. When the technician asks the patient to relax the jaw, the artifact dissipates. Muscle potentials are less than 20 ms, whereas cerebral spike potentials are longer, lasting 20–70 ms.

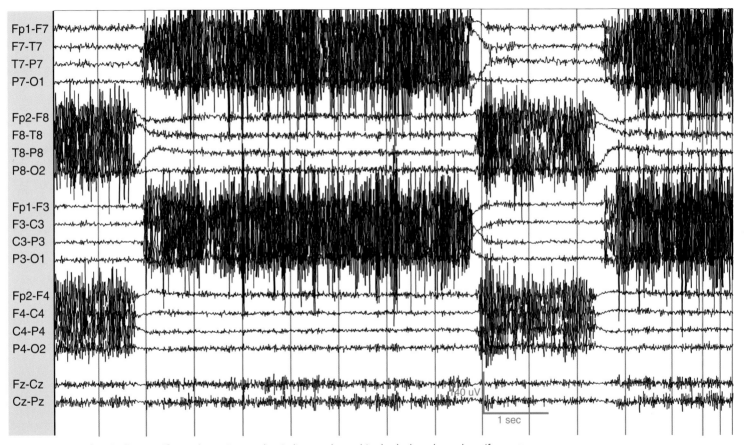

FIGURE 1.25 Tooth-grinding artifact. Alternating tooth grinding produces this checkerboard muscle artifact pattern.

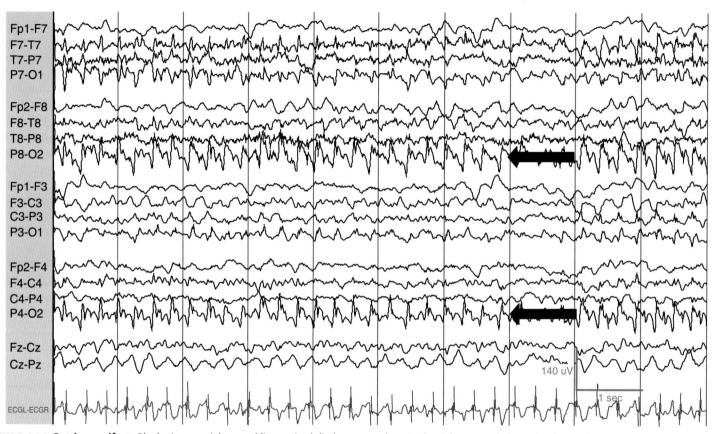

FIGURE 1.26 Patting artifact. Rhythmic potentials resembling an ictal discharge seen here in the right occipital electrodes *(arrows)*, usually produced by a mother who holds her baby on her lap during the EEG. Notice the lack of a field anterior to the artifact.

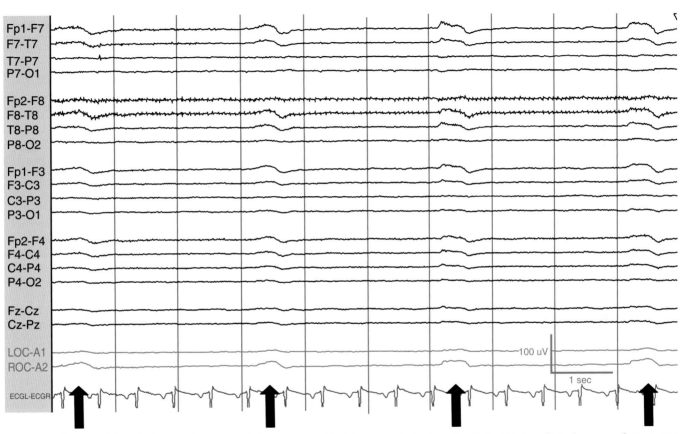

FIGURE 1.27 Ventilator artifact. Wide excursions *(arrows)* that may resemble delta waves. A check on the rhythmicity (usually in the range of 12 per minute), along with a stereotyped waveform, makes the diagnosis. Note that the artifact, in cases where the patient overrides the respirator, may demonstrate irregularity. Amplitude can vary.

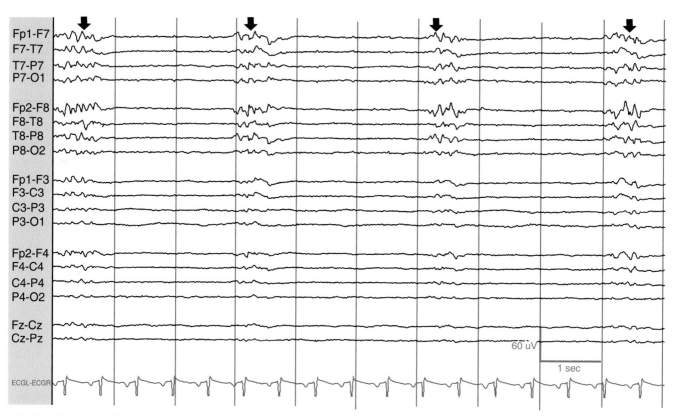

FIGURE 1.28 Respiratory artifact. Note the periodic bursts of sharply contoured theta/alpha frequency activity, prominently seen over the anterior regions. In this patient (same patient as in Fig. 1.27), this activity correlated with the ventilator rate (chest rising movement) and disappeared with suction. This artifact is caused by the movement of fluids within the upper respiratory tract and/or the tube and can also occur irregularly in a patient overriding the respirator. Concomitant use of video and/or audio (sometimes you can hear gurgling sounds) can help to prevent misinterpreting these artifacts as cerebral rhythm.

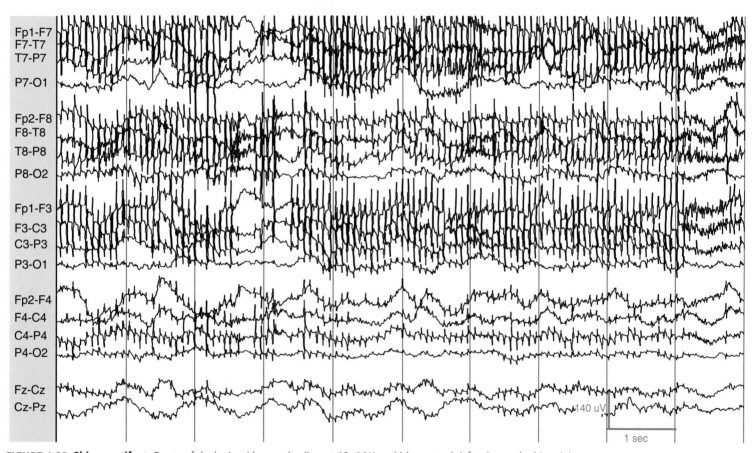

FIGURE 1.29 Shiver artifact. Bursts of rhythmic widespread spikes at 10–14 Hz, which are too brief to be cerebral in origin.

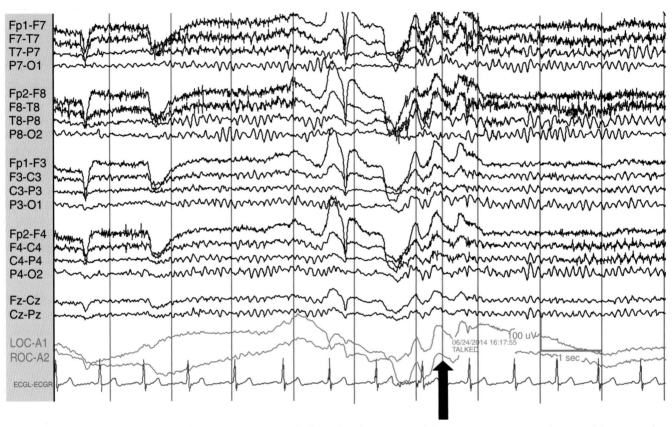

FIGURE 1.30 **Glossokinetic artifact.** The tip of the tongue is negatively charged, and movement of the tongue can cause synchronous delta activity *(arrow)* in the frontal derivations.

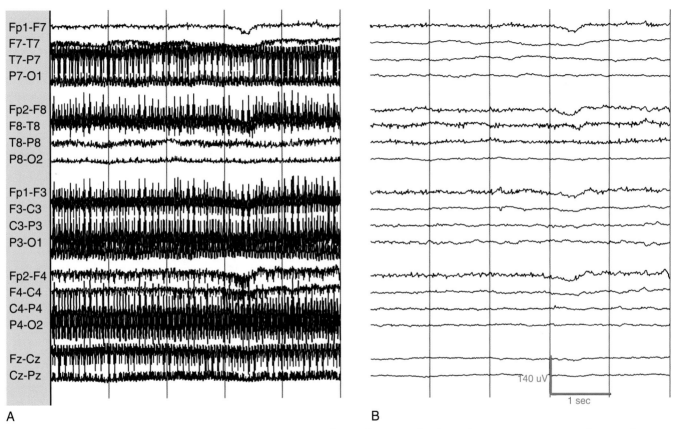

A   B

FIGURE 1.31 60 Hz artifact. Rhythmic frequency at 60 Hz (or 50 Hz in Europe) secondary to nearby electrical apparatus or poor grounding, usually expressed because of high electrode impedance but sometimes (particularly in the ICU) difficult to eliminate. (A) Shows EEG with a great deal of 60 Hz artifact. In (B), the notch filter has been applied.

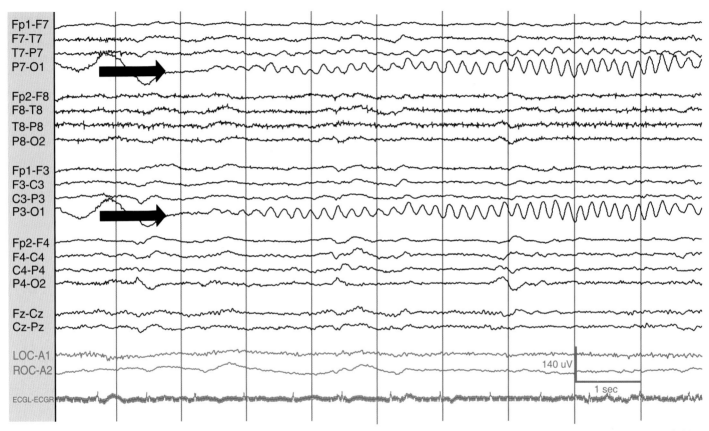

FIGURE 1.32 Tremor artifact. 4–6 Hz tremor artifact *(arrows)* posteriorly in this 66-year-old woman with Parkinson's disease. Note how there is little field anteriorly, which would be very unusual for a cerebrally generated wave.

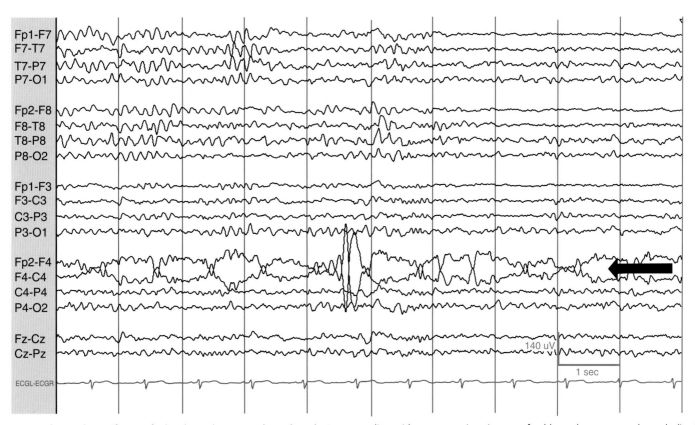

FIGURE 1.33 Electrode artifact. A faulty electrode contact *(arrow)* results in a recording with an exact mirror image referable to the common electrode (in this case, F4). In referential recording, only one channel reflects the discharge. In both cases, there is no potential field. A faulty electrode can also "pop," resulting in a mirror image for only a moment.

Further reading

Adrian, E.D., Matthews, B.H.C., 1934. The Berger rhythm: potential changes from the occipital lobes in man. Brain 57, 355–385.

American Clinical Neurophysiology Society Guidelines. www.acns.org.

Berger, H., 1929. Ueber das elektroenkephalogramm des menschen. Arch. Psychiatr 87, 527–570.

Binnie, C.D., Rowan, A.J., Gutter, T., 1982. A Manual of Electroencephalographic Technology. University Press, Cambridge.

Brittenham, D., 1974. Recognition and reduction of physiological artifacts. Am. J. EEG Technol 14, 158–165.

Buzsáki, G., Traub, R., Pedley, T., 2003. The cellular basis of EEG activity. In: Ebersole, J., Pedley, T.A. (Eds.), Current Practice of Clinical Electroencephalography. Lippincott Williams & Wilkins, Philadelphia, pp. 1–11.

Buzsáki, G., Anastassiou, C., Koch, C., 2012. The origin of extracellular fields and currents—EEG, ECoG, LFP and spikes. Nature Rev. Neurosci. 13, 407–420.

Buzsáki, G., Schomburg, E.W., 2015. What does gamma coherence tell us about interregional neural communication? Nat. Neurosci. 18, 484–489.

Cosandier-Rimélé, D., Bartolomei, F., Merlet, I., Chauvel, P., Wendling, F., 2012. Recording of fast activity at the onset of partial seizures: depth EEG vs. scalp EEG. Neuroimage 59, 3474–3487.

Ebersole, J.S., 2003. Cortical generators and EEG voltage fields. In: Ebersole, J., Pedley, T.A. (Eds.), Current Practice of Clinical Electroencephalography. Lippincott Williams & Wilkins, Philadelphia, pp. 12–31.

Harris, A.Z., Gordon, J.A., 2015. Long-range neural synchrony in behavior. Annu. Rev. Neurosci. 38, 171–194.

Klass, D.W., 1977. Symposium on EEG montages: which, when, why and whither. Introduction. Am. J. EEG Technol 17, 1–3.

Litt, B., Cranstoun, S.D., 2003. Engineering principles. In: Ebersole, J., Pedley, T.A. (Eds.), Current Practice of Clinical Electroencephalography. Lippincott Williams & Wilkins, Philadelphia, pp. 32–71.

Tao, J.X., Ray, A., Hawes-Ebersole, S., Ebersole, J.S., 2005. Intracranial EEG substrates of scalp EEG interictal spikes. Epilepsia 46, 669–676.

Telenczuk, B., Dehghani, N., Le Van Quyen, M., et al., 2017. Local field potentials primarily reflect inhibitory neuron activity in human and monkey cortex. Sci. Rep. 7, 1–10.

THE NORMAL EEG

Understanding the elements of the normal EEG is a prerequisite for developing expertise in interpreting the abnormal record. In the following discussion, the frequency bands and individual waveforms found in the normal adult EEG are described for both the waking and sleeping states.

Alpha activity

Hans Berger, the Berlin psychiatrist who in 1929 recorded the first EEG in humans, described a rhythm in the alpha frequency (8 to <13 Hz) in the posterior regions of the head. This is the posterior dominant rhythm (PDR) (Fig. 2.1). The PDR is of maximal amplitude in the occipital regions and attenuates with eye opening. It is best seen when the person is in the relaxed, waking state with eyes closed.

The PDR is in the alpha frequency in a normal adult. In normal adults, the PDR should be above 8.5 Hz, as the PDR of 8 Hz is only seen in <1% of normal adults at any age.

In assessing the PDR, look for the patient's best—that is, the highest posterior frequency achieved during the most alert state. Slower posterior rhythms in the theta range or theta waves admixed with the alpha may be due to mild drowsiness and thus have no pathological significance.

The PDR is usually symmetric but may be of higher amplitude over the nondominant hemisphere. In that case, a 2 : 1 ratio is acceptable. If the ratio is greater than 2 : 1, it may be related to an abnormality, but it also could be the result of incorrect electrode placement. The latter is more likely if the lower-amplitude alpha is well organized and equally persistent as that on the opposite side. Consideration should be given to the possible presence of an insulating process between the scalp electrodes and the cerebral cortex, as might be seen with a subdural collection. In that case, the alpha on the affected side may either be markedly depressed in amplitude or absent.

The absence of the PDR on one side is always pathological. In older subjects, this asymmetry is often due to remote infarction. In younger subjects, the cause is more likely to be congenital.

The PDR, while usually maximal in the occipital regions, often distributes to the adjacent parietal and posterior temporal areas. Moreover, this may be variable over the course of the recording.

If the PDR increases in frequency when the patient opens their eyes and persists with the eyes open, or appears only during eye opening, drowsiness is a likely cause. When the frequency transiently increases immediately after eye closure, it is called alpha squeak. Some people have little or no PDR during the resting state. This finding has no clinical significance and occurs in perhaps 5% of individuals. If the patient is tense, the PDR may not be recorded. In such cases, the PDR may appear as the patient becomes more relaxed.

Take note of processes that may lead to a decline in PDR frequency. These include (but are not limited to) the effect of antiseizure medication(s) such as phenytoin or valproic acid, sedative medications, early dementias, increased intracranial pressure, CNS infections, hypothyroidism, and other metabolic disorders such as hepatic insufficiency.

Note that waves in the alpha frequency may be found in various locations and in various states (e.g., alpha coma or during a seizure). Such

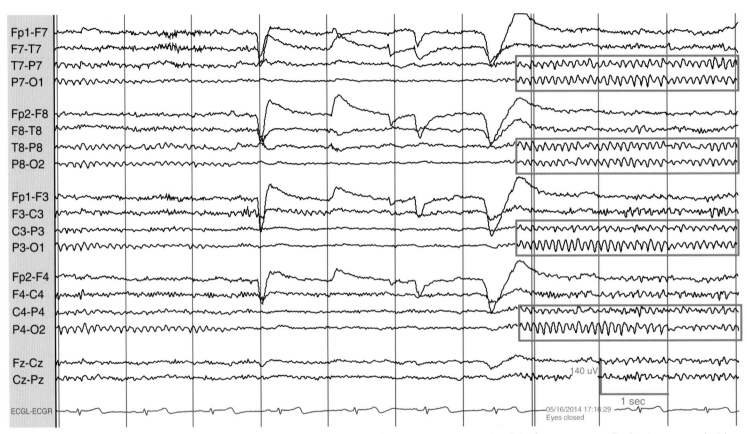

FIGURE 2.1 Posterior dominant rhythm (PDR). Note the sinusoidal rhythm in the posterior regions in the alpha frequency range *(box)*. It is attenuated with eye opening and best seen with eye closure.

waves are not the PDR as described earlier. If a record contains alpha frequency and looks relatively normal, interpretation depends on the state of the patient and the presence of reactivity. In a comatose patient (e.g., after cardiopulmonary arrest), with widespread alpha activity that does not react to eye movements or undergo state change, it is termed alpha coma and carries a poor prognosis.

Beta activity

Beta activity is defined as a frequency in the range of 13 to 30 Hz and is present in the background of most subjects, seen prominently during wakefulness and transitions to drowsiness. If completely absent, it may represent an abnormality, depending on other features of the EEG. Maximal beta amplitude is usually in the frontocentral regions, but it may be widespread. It does not respond to eye opening, as does the PDR. During drowsiness, beta may seem to increase in amplitude. This appears to be a function of amplitude diminution of other background frequencies and thus is more apparent than real.

Beta activity increases in amplitude and abundance by various psychoactive drugs (e.g., barbiturates, chloral hydrate, benzodiazepines, tricyclic antidepressants, and propofol). In these circumstances, the beta activity is usually between 14 and 16 Hz (Fig. 2.2).

Perhaps the most important finding when analyzing beta activity is interhemispheric asymmetry. In particular, the side of reduced amplitude usually points to the pathological hemisphere. Examples include acute and remote infarct, subdural collections, and porencephaly. By the same token, beta amplitude may be unilaterally increased. This occurs in the setting of a previous craniotomy (the so-called breach artifact). In this case, breach refers to an opening or rift (e.g., "Captain, there is a breach in the hull!" versus "Doctor, the baby is breech!"). Lower impedances from the lack of skull continuity result in higher amplitudes of beta activity. Brain abscess, stroke, tumors, vascular malformations, and cortical dysplasia can be associated with either a focal decrease or an enhancement of beta activity. Beta asymmetry, if present, should always be considered in concert with asymmetry of other background frequencies.

Theta activity

Theta activity (4 to <8 Hz) is often present in the waking adult EEG, although it may be completely absent. It tends to be somewhat more evident in the midline and temporal derivations. Approximately 35% of normal young adults show intermittent theta rhythm during relaxed wakefulness that is maximal in the frontocentral head regions. Also, intermittent theta frequency in temporal leads, either bilateral or unilateral (usually left more than right), can be seen in the asymptomatic elderly population with an incidence of about 35%.

If theta activity is consistently found in only one location or is predominant over one hemisphere, it is likely to reflect underlying structural disease. The lesion, however, is usually less malignant, or extensive, than in the case of delta-range focality. Examples are meningioma, low-grade glioma, and remote infarction.

Diffuse theta is usual in children. In the young, theta abundance is quite variable, and one should be flexible when determining whether the theta is excessive or not. When in doubt, err on the side of normality. In comatose patients who have suffered catastrophic brain damage, rhythmic theta may be found diffusely. This finding is termed theta coma.

Delta activity

Delta activity (<4 Hz) was described in 1936 by W. Gray Walter, a young English physiologist. He gathered his bulky EEG apparatus in an operating room where a patient was undergoing neurosurgery for a malignant tumor. Electrodes placed over the involved area recorded very slow, high-voltage potentials that were slower in frequency than previously reported waveforms. Walter termed these potentials delta waves. Since

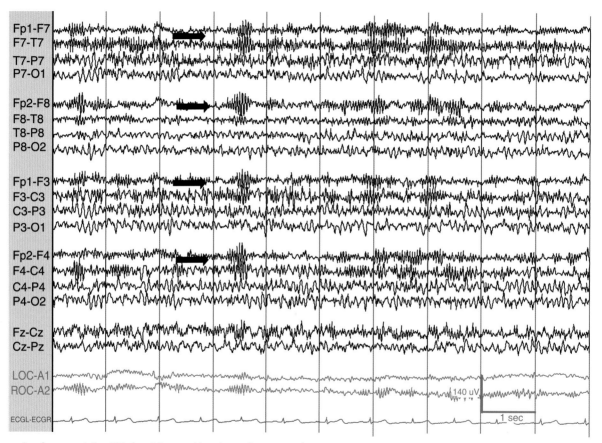

FIGURE 2.2 Excessive beta activity. This is a 30-year-old male on clonazepam for anxiety. The beta activity is best seen over the frontal electrodes *(arrows)*.

that time, focal delta activity has proved a reliable indicator of localized disease of the brain.

As a rule, delta waves are not present in the adult during wakefulness. It follows that their presence in wake implies cerebral dysfunction. Delta waves are a normal and important component of adult sleep.

There are other circumstances wherein delta is a normal component of the EEG. For instance, delta is prominent in infants and young children and is common in adolescents in the posterior head regions (posterior slow waves of youth).

Excessive diffuse delta is abnormal and indicates encephalopathy of nonspecific etiology. Focal polymorphic delta activity usually indicates a structural lesion involving the white matter, especially when it is continuously seen. Focal rhythmic delta activity can involve the ipsilateral gray matter, be indicative of underlying cortical hyperexcitability, and indicates a tendency to have seizures from that area.

Features of sleep

Often, the easiest way to tell if someone is drowsy is by the absence of eye blinks. Drowsiness or N1 sleep is characterized by slowing, fragmentation (increasing irregularity), and ultimate disappearance of the PDR. The background may appear to be generally of lower voltage (due to absence of the PDR), and beta activity may be more obvious. Diffuse theta activity appears and increases in abundance. Vertex waves, which appear during N1, are synchronous, episodic, sharply contoured potentials (<200 ms in duration) that are maximal over the central regions. They may assume a very sharp, spike like configuration; are variable in amplitude; and sometimes occur in rhythmic runs. In addition, positive occipital sharp transients of sleep (POSTs) may be quite prominent. These potentials have the appearance of sharp waves, are electropositive at the occipital electrodes, and may be mono- or biphasic in configuration. POSTs are often bilaterally synchronous and found more commonly in young and

middle-aged adults. Do not be surprised to find long rhythmic runs of POSTs that could be mistaken by the unwary for an ictal discharge (Fig. 2.3). Both vertex waves and POSTs may persist into N2 sleep.

N2 sleep arrives with the appearance of well-defined sleep spindles and K-complexes (Fig. 2.4). Sleep spindles are synchronous, sinusoidal waves at 12–14 ($\pm$2) Hz with a potential maximum in the central regions. If spindles are only fragmentary or very brief, the patient is not considered to be firmly in N2. K-complexes are high-voltage (>200 μV), synchronous bi- or triphasic slow potentials (>500 ms) usually with a central or bifrontal preponderance, often (but not invariably) in close association with sleep spindles. A K-complex can be evoked by a sudden auditory stimulus (e.g., a K-complex can occur when the technician **K**nocks).

N3 sleep (slow-wave sleep) is characterized by increasing amounts of diffuse delta activity, occupying more than 20% of the background (Fig. 2.5). At the same time, there is a progressive decline in sleep spindles—in fact, they usually disappear. The delta may reach very high voltage without clinical significance. In adults, N3 is seldom encountered during routine recording.

Rapid eye movement (REM) sleep is characterized by rapid eye movements and loss of muscle tone (Fig. 2.6). The EEG background consists of low-voltage theta activity, and eye channels demonstrate irregular vertical and horizontal eye movements. Epileptiform discharges are seldom present in REM sleep. Non-REM sleep and REM sleep alternate in cycles 4–6 times during normal sleep, with increasing REM sleep in the last third of the night. Recall that the first REM period usually occurs about 90 minutes after sleep onset, and patients with narcolepsy experience REM at sleep onset. However, a routine EEG with REM may reflect sleep deprivation and does not necessarily mean a sleep disorder such as narcolepsy.

The recording of sleep is one of the most powerful diagnostic adjuncts in electroencephalography. Relatively minor abnormalities

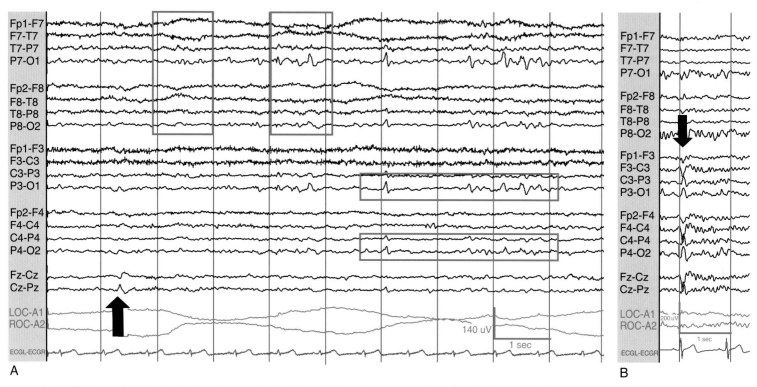

FIGURE 2.3 N1 sleep. (A) Note the lack of the posterior dominant rhythm, relative attenuation of the background with more low-voltage fast activity anteriorly, slow horizontal roving eye movements (*first vertical box:* eyes to the left, *second vertical box:* eyes to the right), appearance of subtle vertex wave *(arrow)*, and positive occipital sharp transients of sleep (POSTs) *(horizontal boxes)*. (B) A well-formed vertex wave *(arrow)* with phase reversal at the C_z, C_3, and C_4 electrodes.

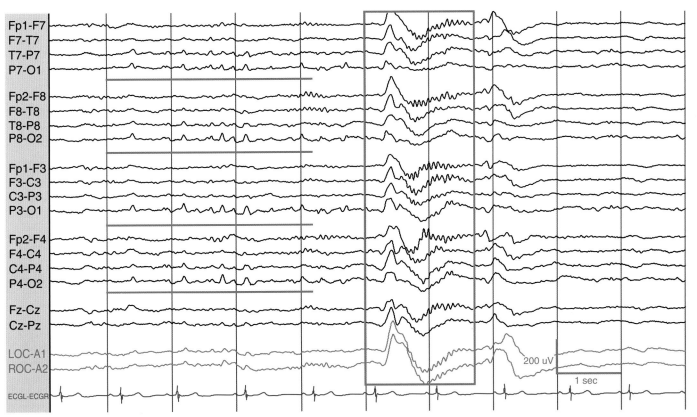

FIGURE 2.4 N2 sleep. N2 sleep is characterized by the appearance of K-complexes and sleep spindles *(box)*. K-complexes are bifrontally or centrally predominant diffuse high-voltage, synchronous slow potentials (>500 ms). Sleep spindles often follow the K-complexes. Note runs of positive occipital sharp transients of sleep (POSTs) preceding the K-complex and spindles *(underline)*.

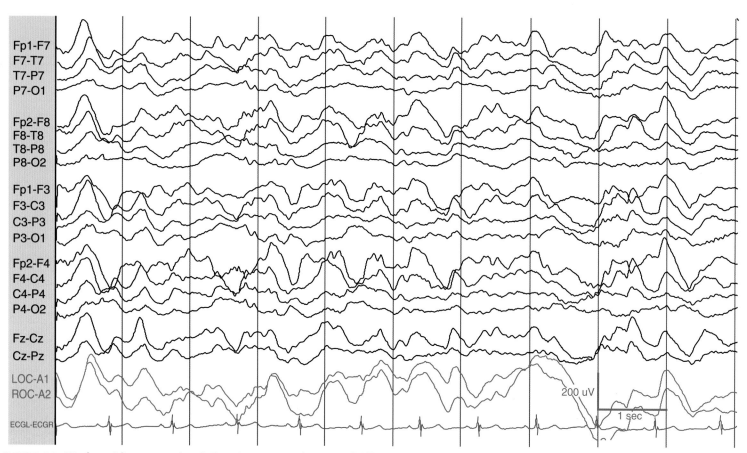

FIGURE 2.5 N3 sleep (slow-wave sleep). There is an increased amount of diffuse delta activity and decreased sleep spindles.

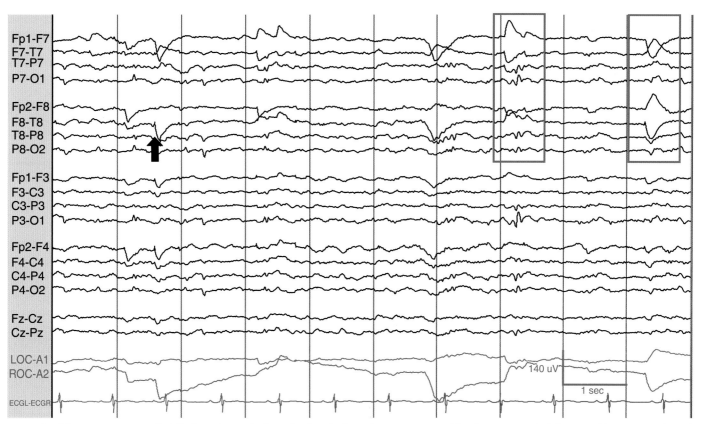

FIGURE 2.6 Rapid eye movement (REM) sleep. Note the irregular, fast, horizontal eye movements (*first box:* eyes to the left, *second box:* eyes to the right. Trick: you can tell the direction of the eye movements by imagining an eyeball fitting into the oval shape). They sometimes seem spiky *(arrow)*, which represents artifacts of the lateral rectus muscles.

on the routine EEG may be amplified during sleep, and new abnormalities may appear. This is particularly the case in epileptiform activity. Most patients become drowsy at some point during a routine recording, and many actually sleep spontaneously for variable periods. In patients with focal epilepsy, focal spike or sharp wave discharges often appear or are increased during N1 (drowsiness) and N2 sleep. Likewise, focal slow-wave abnormalities may be exaggerated during these stages. With deeper sleep (N3), there is a tendency for epileptiform activity and focal slowing to become less obvious.

SPECIAL CONSIDERATIONS IN THE ELDERLY

The EEG in the elderly, regardless of age, can be normal in every regard. This extends to the PDR, which may maintain a steady 10 Hz frequency throughout life. Alternatively, there may be a gradual decline in the frequency of the PDR. A specific disease process may not be evident, but the slower PDR probably reflects a degree of cerebral dysfunction (e.g., cerebrovascular disease or a degenerative process). The PDR is not reported as abnormal until it falls below 8.5 Hz. Beta activity may decrease in the elderly. Another common finding is intermittent bitemporal theta and delta activity, symmetric or asymmetric, perhaps preponderant on one side. Temporal theta is generally considered normal if it occurs in <15% of the record. Temporal delta waves probably represent underlying cerebral pathology (e.g., cerebrovascular disease). However, there may be no focal abnormality on an imaging study. We emphasize this because the ordering clinician should be aware that such a patient is relatively unlikely to have a brain tumor or stroke.

Generalized rhythmic delta activity (GRDA) with a frontal predominance is a normal finding in elderly drowsiness. This feature may have no specific significance. It is possible that frontally predominant GRDA may represent some degree of subcortical dysfunction secondary to vascular disease or other degenerative factors. It is not, however, particularly helpful in making a specific diagnosis, and it is not necessary to call it abnormal in a report.

Sleep features in the elderly tend to be less well defined than those encountered in younger adults. Sleep spindles may be more irregular or of lower voltage. Similarly, vertex sharp waves may be less well defined. REM sleep is preserved in aging. However, the abundance of N3 sleep diminishes with age.

ACTIVATION PROCEDURES

Hyperventilation (HV)

HV is a standard procedure during routine EEG recording. It is thought that the usefulness of HV depends on vasoconstriction secondary to the resultant decreased CO_2 concentration, thus inducing relative cerebral ischemia and decreased glucose utilization. Subjects may complain of lightheadedness or tingling in the extremities. Even tetany secondary to hypocalcemia may occur with particularly vigorous HV. The procedure is most effective in the young; in the elderly, it has little effect.

The standard response is moderate to high voltage, often rhythmic, delta and theta slowing with bifrontal preponderance (Fig. 2.7). In the young, nearly continuous delta may be evoked. HV may bring out epileptiform discharges and focal slowing (Fig. 2.8). In unmedicated children with absence epilepsy, it may provoke an absence seizure. As a rule, HV is carried out for 3 minutes with vigorous exhalation at an increased but not particularly rapid rate. Rapid HV moves little air and has correspondingly little effect. After the conclusion of HV, the record should return to baseline levels in about 1 minute. If return to baseline occurs after a protracted period, it may represent an abnormality. The classic cause of a long return to baseline is hypoglycemia.

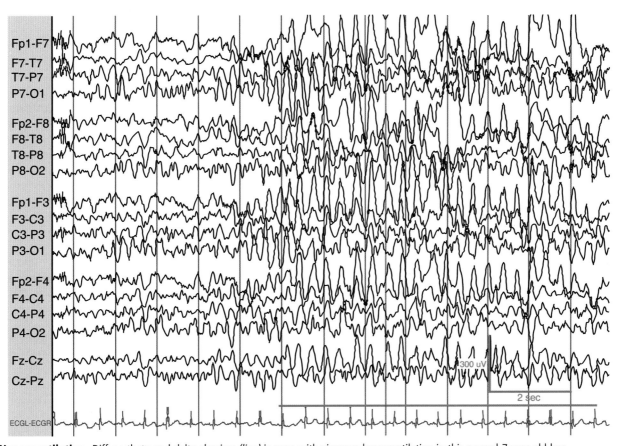

FIGURE 2.7 Hyperventilation. Diffuse theta and delta slowing *(line)* is seen with vigorous hyperventilation in this normal 7-year-old boy.

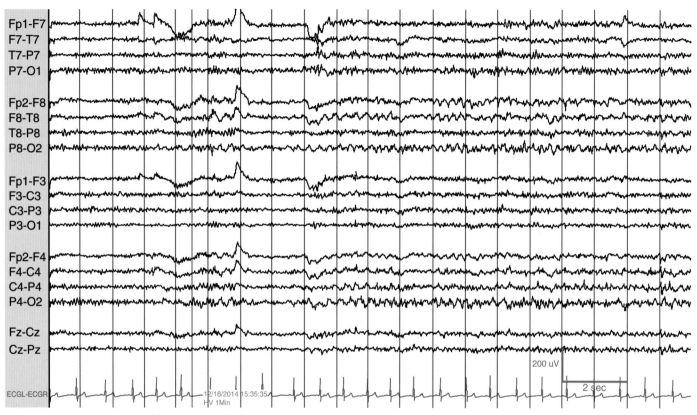

FIGURE 2.8 Focal slowing induced by hyperventilation: A 36-year-old woman with a normal brain MRI and focal epilepsy. Right hemispheric slowing was seen with hyperventilation. The rest of the EEG showed occasional polymorphic right frontotemporal slowing.

HV is often omitted in subjects over the age of 65 years due to its low yield. An elderly person's vascular system is less responsive to the metabolic changes precipitated by HV. In cases of suspected epilepsy, however, HV may be useful despite these limitations. Note that there are few contraindications for performing HV. In general, it is not performed in patients with pulmonary and cardiac diseases. HV may be performed in patients with brain tumors, although if the resting record reveals clear focal slowing, the procedure probably offers little additional information.

Photic stimulation (PS)

PS is another standard procedure during routine EEG recording. This procedure is easily carried out with strobe units that flash for 5–10 seconds at frequencies typically between 1 and 35 Hz. PS can evoke a rhythmic frequency in the occipital derivations termed photic driving (Fig. 2.9). If the response to the flash train is 1:1, it is termed the fundamental. It is not unusual to see harmonic (twice the flash frequency) and/or subharmonic (half the flash frequency) responses. Often, there is no change in frequency in the occipital derivations during PS. This has no pathological significance. If photic driving is absent on one side, it may support a diagnosis of unilateral structural disease involving the occipital region (e.g., infarction in posterior cerebral artery territory). Rarely, individuals have a photomyogenic response, with myogenic potentials seen in the frontal derivations, which are time locked to the flash frequency (Fig. 2.10). This is not an epileptiform abnormality!

The major utility of the procedure is in patients with epilepsy suspected of having seizures precipitated by flickering light. There are various degrees of photosensitivity, the most prominent being a synchronous high-voltage spike/polyspike-wave discharge. This phenomenon is called the photoparoxysmal response (Fig. 2.11). Photosensitivity is often maximal at 14–16 flashes per second. Some patients demonstrate a photoparoxysmal response at a specific frequency or a very narrow frequency band. For patients with a marked degree of photosensitivity, an abnormal response may be obtained over a wide frequency range. Note that the technician must stop the flash train if generalized polyspike-wave bursts occur. If the stimulus is continued, a generalized seizure may result. Typically, the evoked discharges outlast cessation of the flash stimulus by a second or so.

Sleep deprivation

Sleep deprivation is a powerful activator of epileptiform activity. It is sometimes suggested that the subject stay up all night before the appointment the next morning, but a brief period of sleep may be permitted. The patient is instructed to stay up late, sleep for 1 or 2 hours, and then come to the EEG laboratory for testing in the morning. No caffeinated beverages are permitted, as the goal is to have the patient sleep for a portion of the recording. HV and PS are carried out early in the test, after which the patient is allowed to sleep. One can expect an increase in or de novo appearance of focal epileptiform activity in about 30% of patients with epilepsy. Sleep deprivation is often used during a video EEG admission in order to increase the probability of capturing the patient's typical seizure.

NORMAL VARIANTS AND PAROXYSMAL PHENOMENA OF UNCERTAIN SIGNIFICANCE

Alpha variants

Slow alpha variant appears in the occipital regions at a frequency one-half that of the ongoing PDR. Suspect its presence when PDR activity has a notched appearance, revealing its subharmonic relationship. Slow alpha variant has the same characteristics as the PDR itself—for example, it attenuates with eye opening. Fast alpha variant also appears in the occipital areas and has a frequency twice that of the usual PDR (Fig. 2.12).

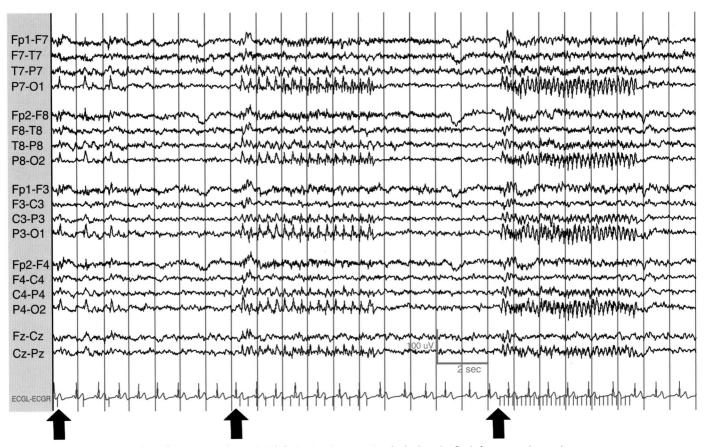

FIGURE 2.9 Photic driving. Rhythmic frequency in the occipital derivations is seen, time-locked to the flash frequency *(arrows)*.

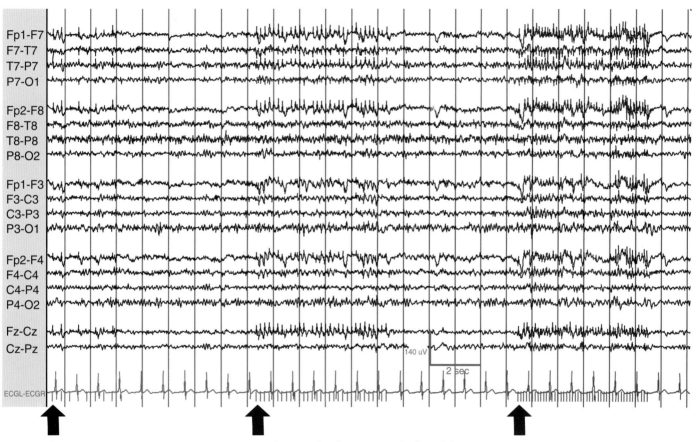

FIGURE 2.10 Photomyogenic response: Myogenic potentials (EMG artifacts) are seen in the frontal derivations, time-locked to the flash frequency *(arrows)*.

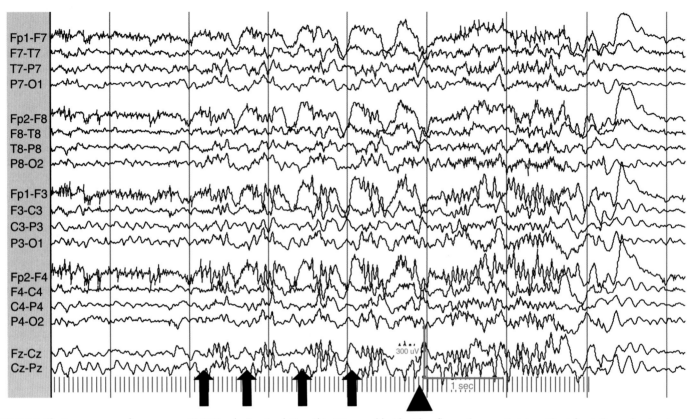

FIGURE 2.11 Photoparoxysmal response. At 17 Hz photic stimulation, this 18-year-old girl with reflex epilepsy gets intermittent frontally predominant polyspikes *(arrows)*, followed by a 2-second run of polyspikes *(arrowhead)*. She typically finds this pleasurable (at home will self-induce in front of the TV) and is not compliant with medication.

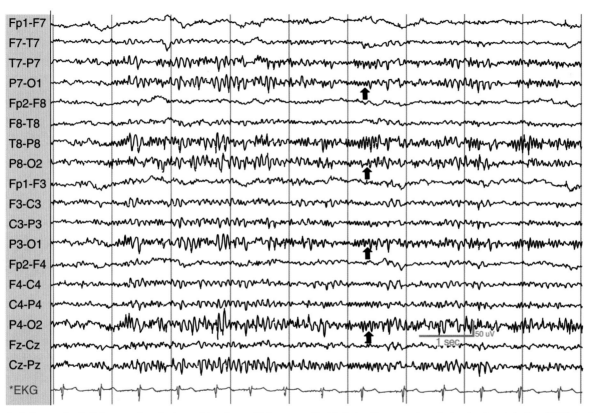

FIGURE 2.12 Fast alpha variant. This normal variant consists of a rapid frequency that is twice the normal posterior dominant rhythm (PDR). In this case, the variant is prominent in the posterior quadrants at a frequency of 20 Hz. It has the same general characteristics as the alpha (e.g., attenuation with eye opening).

These variants may alternate with the standard PDR, or the standard PDR may not be present at all. Both are normal.

Mu rhythm

Mu rhythm is arch-shaped alpha frequency found in the central derivations (C3/C4) over the motor strip (Fig. 2.13). It may be unilateral or bilateral; if bilateral, it may be synchronous or asynchronous. Mu is sometimes more evident during drowsiness and when the eyes are open. It is considered to be the resting rhythm of the rolandic cortex. Mu attenuates with movement of the opposite upper limb (e.g., making a fist). Interestingly, even the thought of moving the opposite limb can attenuate the mu rhythm. It is often prominent over the site of a craniotomy. The importance of mu lies mainly in its recognition as a normal finding.

Lambda waves

Lambda waves are electropositive transients in the occipital regions (Fig. 2.14). They are sharply contoured, usually symmetric and synchronous, and can be mistaken for epileptiform potentials. At the same time, lambda often goes unnoticed due to lack of awareness by the reader, as well as the absence of circumstances, which lead to their expression, namely scanning eye movements. Having the subject look at a picture containing interesting subjects or details may provoke lambda waves. Lambda waves probably represent visual evoked potentials. Again, the principal advantage to recognizing lambda is the knowledge that it is a normal finding and not an example of epileptiform activity.

Rhythmic midtemporal theta discharge (RMTD)

This was formerly known as psychomotor variant. RMTD consists of rhythmic, sharply contoured theta waves at 5–6 Hz in the midtemporal regions (Fig. 2.15). The bursts are brief, usually 1 second or so in duration, and may be unilateral or independent in both midtemporal regions. This phenomenon

appears during drowsiness and has no clear clinical significance. Incidentally, psychomotor variant (the old term) was meant to suggest that this phenomenon might be correlated with focal seizures with impaired awareness (formerly psychomotor seizures). In fact, this usually does not turn out to be the case. The exception occurs when there are coexisting epileptiform discharges or seizures in a similar location in the same patient.

Wicket spikes

Wicket spikes are sharply contoured rhythmic frequencies varying from 7 to 11 Hz, maximal in the midtemporal derivations, occurring in isolation or in brief runs (Fig. 2.16). Wicket spikes are usually seen in adults, and look like a comb or wicket fence. At times, one of the waves may stand out from the others, giving the appearance of a sharp wave or a spike. In wicket spikes, the duration of the waveforms is similar, regardless of variations in amplitude. Unlike epileptiform sharp waves or spikes, there is no aftergoing slow wave. This finding occurs during drowsiness and has no apparent clinical significance. The reader should compare the locations of wicket spikes and mu rhythm (the latter is found in the central regions).

Subclinical rhythmic electroencephalographic discharges of adults (SREDA)

SREDA masquerades as an electrographic seizure in one or both hemispheres (Fig. 2.17). Unlike most other benign variants that occur more in young adults in a drowsy state, this pattern typically occurs in the older population (over 50 years of age) and is seen during waking and sleeping. It is typically maximal at the temporoparietal junction but can be seen at the vertex as well. It may appear in two forms: (1) symmetric or asymmetric bilateral bursts of rhythmic sharply contoured theta activity; or (2) sudden appearance of repetitive sharp or slow waveforms that become shorter in interval that mimics the evolution of an electrographic

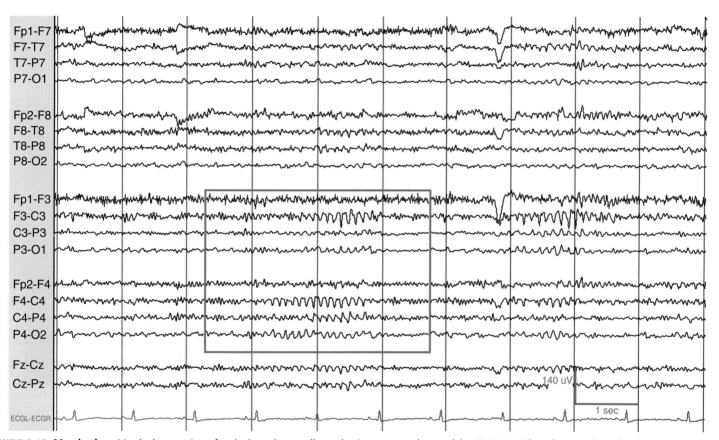

FIGURE 2.13 Mu rhythm. Mu rhythm consists of arch-shaped, centrally predominant waves *(rectangle)* at 7–11 Hz. When the contralateral arm is moved, mu rhythm will attenuate. In fact, if the subject even thinks about moving an arm (say the right arm), mu rhythm will attenuate on the left.

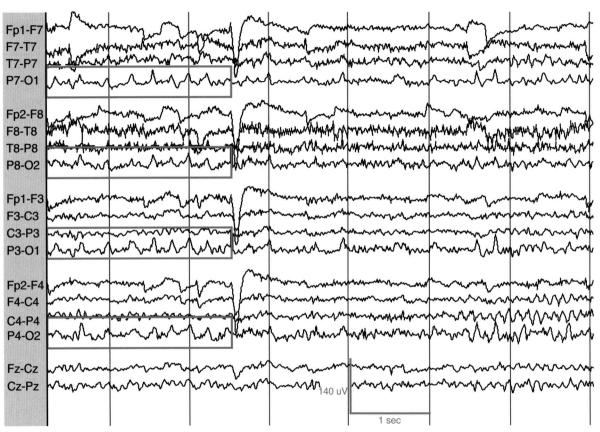

FIGURE 2.14 Lambda waves. Lambda waves *(boxes)* are sharp transients recorded in the occipital region (positive at O1/O2; negative at P7/P8/P3/P4), induced in the waking state by scanning the environment.

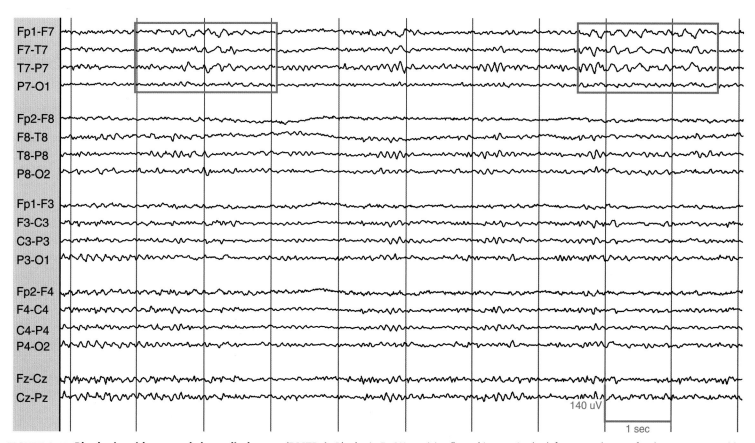

FIGURE 2.15 Rhythmic midtemporal theta discharges (RMTDs). Rhythmic 5–6 Hz activity *(boxes)* is seen in the left temporal area of a drowsy 44-year-old woman who was hospitalized for new-onset psychogenic nonepileptic attacks. This woman had bilateral abundant RMTDs. RMTDs are a normal variant.

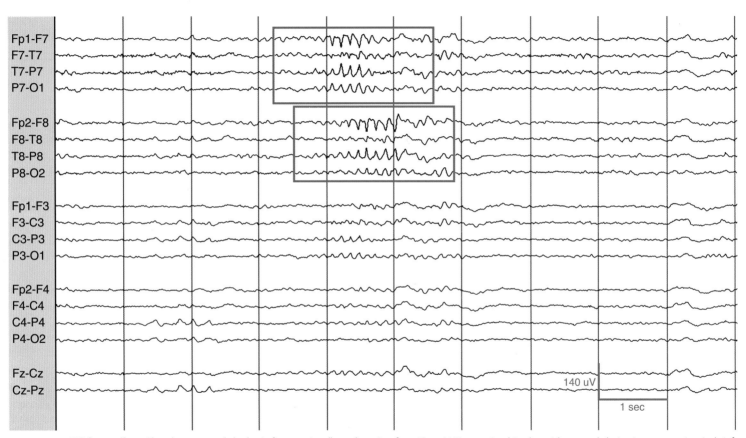

FIGURE 2.16 Wicket spikes. Sharply contoured rhythmic frequencies *(boxes)* varying from 7 to 11 Hz, maximal in the midtemporal derivations, occurring in brief runs. The duration of the waveforms is similar and there is no aftergoing slow wave. Wicket spikes are normal.

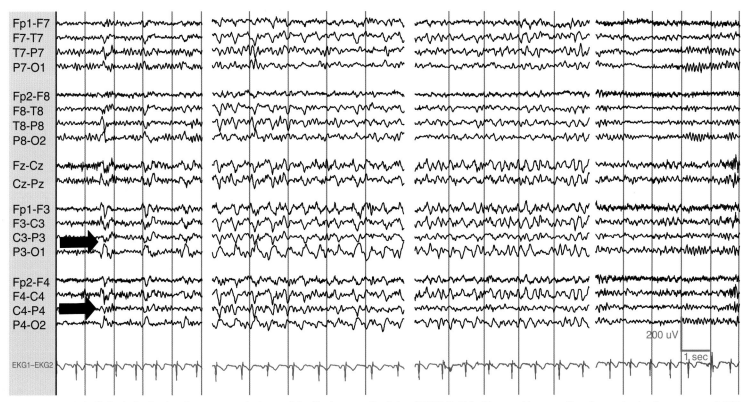

FIGURE 2.17 **Subclinical rhythmic electroencephalographic discharge of adults (SREDA).** This 58-year-old man suffered an episode of syncope, and EEGs showed multiple episodes of SREDA with sharply contoured bilateral temporoparietal delta *(arrows)* that became closer in interval and then resolved with no clinical correlate. He was erroneously treated with antiseizure medications (ASMs), which had no impact on the pattern. He has been off ASMs for several years and has not had any clinical episodes, though this pattern persists.

seizure, followed by a sustained burst that does not continue to evolve. SREDA usually lasts 40–80 seconds and is not followed by postictal slowing. During this time, the patient has no alteration of awareness and is fully responsive. SREDA has no known significance beyond the fact that it must be recognized in order to avoid misdiagnosis.

Small sharp spikes (SSSs)

SSSs are low-amplitude, rapid spikes (Fig. 2.18). They appear in both hemispheres as synchronous or asynchronous, most often in the temporal derivations, and become evident during drowsiness and N2 sleep. They are not thought to be associated with epilepsy. SSSs are also known as benign epileptiform transients of sleep (BETS).

Phantom spike-wave discharges

Phantom spike waves are usually synchronous discharges at a frequency of 5–6 Hz appearing symmetrically (Fig. 2.19). They can have either an anterior or a posterior predominance. The spike itself is usually less prominent than the following slow wave (thus called "phantom" due to the low-amplitude spikes buried within the bursts). The amplitude is often low, with the spike component usually <40 µV and slow wave <50 µV. Spikes appear individually or in brief rhythmic runs and do not have known epileptogenic significance. Higher amplitude of the spikes, anterior predominance, and a slower rate is more likely associated with seizures.

14 and 6 (14/6) positive spikes

14 and 6 positive spikes, as the name implies, are positive in polarity (the range may vary a little, typically 13–17 Hz and 5–7 Hz). They are usually maximal in the posterior quadrants and appear in isolation or in groups (Fig. 2.20). They may be unilateral or bilateral. The two frequencies are often admixed, but one may predominate. They are most commonly seen between 8 and 14 years of age and decrease in adolescence. The phenomenon appears during drowsiness and is best recorded with crossed ear references (essentially wide interelectrode distances). In the past, 14/6 was thought to be associated with a wide variety of conditions, including psychiatric disorders and epilepsy. Although there remains some disagreement as to their significance, they have no known relationship to epilepsy.

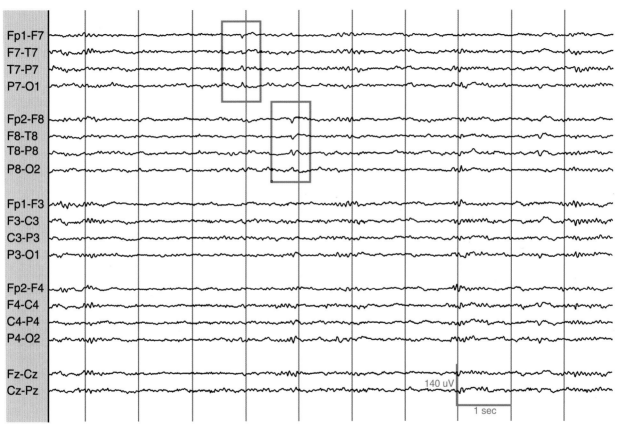

FIGURE 2.18 Small sharp spikes (SSSs). Low-amplitude, asynchronous bilateral temporally maximal rapid spikes *(rectangles)*, seen here in N2 sleep. These are not associated with epilepsy.

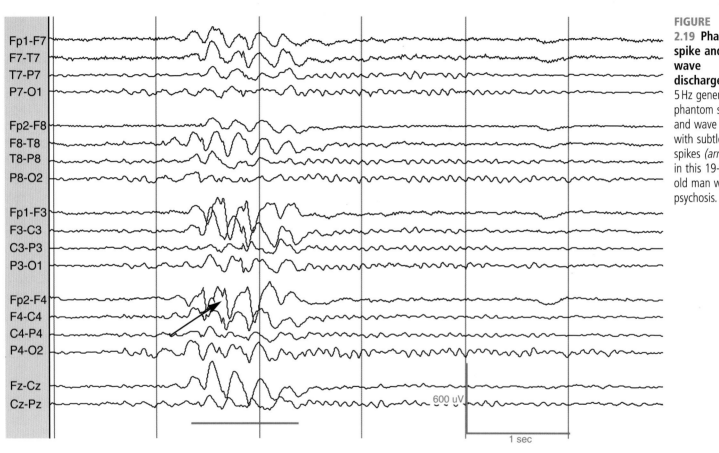

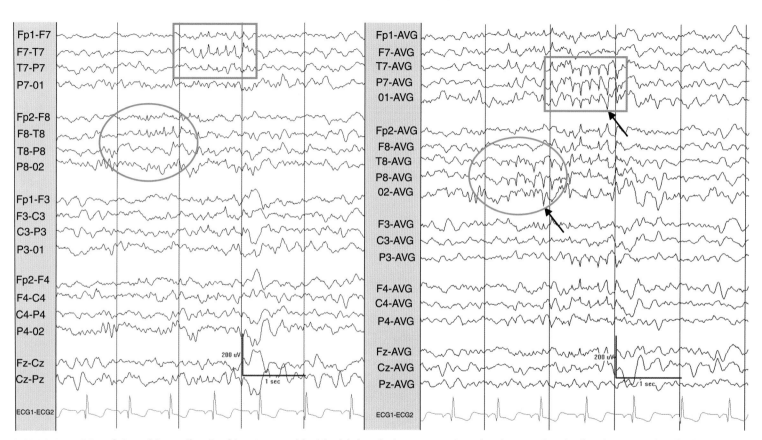

FIGURE 2.20 14 and 6 positive spikes in this 10-year-old girl with headaches. 14 Hz admixed with 6 Hz spikes *(oval)* and 6–7 Hz spikes *(box)* are seen in the temporal regions (in bipolar montage). These are positive in polarity *(arrows)* in the average montage, maximal in the posterior quadrant.

Further reading

Binnie, C.D., Coles, P.A., Margerison, J.H., 1969. The influence of end-tidal carbon dioxide tension on EEG changes during routine hyperventilation in different age groups. Electroencephalogr. Clin. Neurophysiol. 27 (3), 304–306.

Dement, W., Kleitman, N., 1957. Cyclic variations in EEG during sleep and their relation to eye movements, body motility, and dreaming. Electroencephalogr. Clin. Neurophysiol. 9 (4), 673–690.

Erwin, C.W., Somerville, E.R., Radtke, R.A., 1984. A review of electroencephalographic features of normal sleep. J. Clin. Neurophysiol 1 (3), 253–274.

Fountain, N.B., Kim, J.S., Lee, S.I., 1998. Sleep deprivation activates epileptiform discharges independent of the activating effects of sleep. J. Clin. Neurophysiol 15 (1), 69–75.

Gabor, A.J., Seyal, M., 1986. Effect of sleep on the electrographic manifestations of epilepsy. J. Clin. Neurophysiol 3 (1), 23–38.

Gloor, P., Tsai, C., Haddad, F., 1958. An assessment of the value of sleep-electroencephalography for the diagnosis of temporal lobe epilepsy. Electroencephalogr. Clin. Neurophysiol. 10 (4), 633–648.

Hartikainen, P., Soininen, H., Partanen, J., et al., 1992. Aging and spectral analysis of EEG in normal subjects: a link to memory and CSF AChE. Acta. Neurol. Scand 86, 148–155.

Heppenstall, M.E., 1944. The relation between the effects of the blood sugar levels and hyperventilation on the electroencephalogram. J. Neurol. Neurosurg. Psychiatr 7 (3–4), 112–118.

Hubbard, O., Sunde, D., Goldensohn, E.S., 1976. The EEG in centenarians. Electroencephalogr. Clin. Neurophysiol. 40 (4), 407–417.

Hughes, J.R., 1960. Usefulness of photic stimulation in routine clinical electroencephalography. Neurology 10, 777–782.

Hughes, J.R., Cayaffa, J.J., 1977. The EEG in patients at different ages without organic cerebral disease. Electroencephalogr. Clin. Neurophysiol. 42 (6), 776–784.

Klass, D.W., Brenner, R.P., 1995. Electroencephalography of the elderly. J. Clin. Neurophysiol 12 (2), 116–131.

Klass, D.W., Westmoreland, B.F., 1985. Nonepileptogenic epileptiform electroencephalographic activity. Ann. Neurol. 18 (6), 627–635.

Kozelka, J.W., Pedley, T.A., 1990. Beta and mu rhythms. J. Clin. Neurophysiol 7 (2), 191–207.

Lipman, I.J., Hughes, J.R., 1969. Rhythmic mid-temporal discharges. An electro-clinical study. Electroencephalogr. Clin. Neurophysiol 27 (1), 43–47.

Markand, O.N., 1990. Alpha rhythms. J. Clin. Neurophysiol 7 (2), 163–189.

O'Brien, T.J., Sharbrough, F.W., Westmoreland, B.F., et al., 1998. Subclinical rhythmic electrographic discharges of adults (SREDA) revisited: a study using digital EEG analysis. J. Clin. Neurophysiol 15 (6), 493–501.

Patel, V.M., Maulsby, R.L., 1987. How hyperventilation alters the electroencephalogram: a review of controversial viewpoints emphasizing neurophysiological mechanisms. J. Clin. Neurophysiol 4 (2), 101–120.

Reiher, J., Lebel, M., 1977. Wicket spikes: clinical correlates of a previously undescribed EEG pattern. Can. J. Neurol. Sci. 4 (1), 39–47.

Reilly, E.L., Peters, J.F., 1973. Relationship of some varieties of electroencephalographic photosensitivity to clinical convulsive disorders. Neurology 23 (10), 1050–1057.

Tatum, W.O., Husain, A.M., Benbadis, S.R., et al., 2006. Normal adult EEG and patterns of uncertain significance. J. Clin. Neurophysiol 23 (3), 194–207.

Thomas, J.E., Klass, D.W., 1968. Six-per-second spike-and-wave pattern in the electroencephalogram. A reappraisal of its clinical significance. Neurology 18 (6), 587–593.

Westmoreland, B.F., Klass, D.W., 1986. Midline theta rhythm. Arch. Neurol. 43 (2), 139–141.

Westmoreland, B.F., Klass, D.W., 1997. Unusual variants of subclinical rhythmic electrographic discharge of adults (SREDA). Electroencephalogr. Clin. Neurophysiol. 102 (1), 1–4.

Westmoreland, B.F., Reiher, J., Klass, D.W., 1979. Recording small sharp spikes with depth electroencephalography. Epilepsia 20 (6), 599–606.

White, J.C., Langston, J.W., Pedley, T.A., 1977. Benign epileptiform transients of sleep. Clarification of the small sharp spike controversy. Neurology 27 (11), 1061–1068.

The normal EEG from neonates to adolescents 3

NEONATES

Neonatal EEGs are perhaps the most challenging for the student and even for the experienced electroencephalographer. In the neonatal period, the brain is developing rapidly. Within the first 24 weeks of gestation, the cortical layers of the brain form, with migration of neurons and glial cells from the periventricular germinal zone to the cortex. From 24 weeks to term, the brain goes from having a smooth surface to having the intricate pattern of sulcation characteristic of the adult brain. Myelination occurs almost exclusively after birth. Not surprisingly, these changes all impact the neonatal EEG.

For this reason, the electroencephalographer must know the postmenstrual age (PMA) of the neonate. The PMA is the sum of the gestational age (the number of weeks since the last menstrual cycle) and the legal age (age since time of birth). Term newborns are 37–44 weeks PMA, preterm newborns are <37 weeks PMA, and postterm newborns 44–48 weeks PMA. What is normal for a 26-week-old premature infant represents severe cerebral dysfunction for a full-term infant. Persistence or reappearance of a premature pattern for the PMA is a sign of dysmaturity or cerebral dysfunction.

In addition, the neonatal study ideally includes several other recordings to help ascertain the behavioral state of the neonate as well as to assess for apnea. These include electrodes to measure eye movements and muscle tone (with a submental or chin electrode), transducers to measure airflow (a nasal thermistor) and respiratory effort (a thoracic strain gauge). As with adults, in central apnea, there is no activity in either the thoracic strain gauge or nasal thermistor. There is no breathing in central apnea because there is no effort to breathe. In contrast, with obstructive apnea, there is no flow in the nasal thermistor as air is not able to enter, but there is effort in the thoracic strain gauge.

Due to the small head size of the neonate, a reduced 11-contact electrode array is used (Fp1, T7, O1, C3, Fp2, T8, O2, C4, Fz, Cz, Pz). The neonatal EEG is typically read with a time base of 15 mm/second as opposed to 30 mm/second in adult EEGs. This compresses the data of the neonate and facilitates evaluation of continuity and symmetry.

As with all complex analyses, we recommend a systematic approach to the evaluation of the neonatal EEG. Specifically-continuity, symmetry, graphoelements, sleep/wake cycles, and reactivity should be examined for each neonatal EEG (Table 3.1).

Continuity

The normal EEG evolution is one of persistent discontinuity in the premature infant to one of continuity in a fully mature infant. A premature infant of less than 29 weeks PMA may have an EEG that is flat, with medium to high amplitude bursts (50–300 µV) and with an interburst interval (IBI) that can be up to 60 seconds. Between 29 and 32 weeks PMA, IBI is typically 5–8 seconds but can be as long as 30 seconds. The amplitude of the IBI is less than 25 µV. This pattern is known as tracé discontinu (Fig. 3.1). Rare periods of continuous activity may be seen in wake and active sleep. Between 32 and 35 weeks PMA, the IBI becomes shorter and is rarely greater than 10 seconds. At this time, continuous activity may be seen in wake and in active sleep. At 35 weeks PMA,

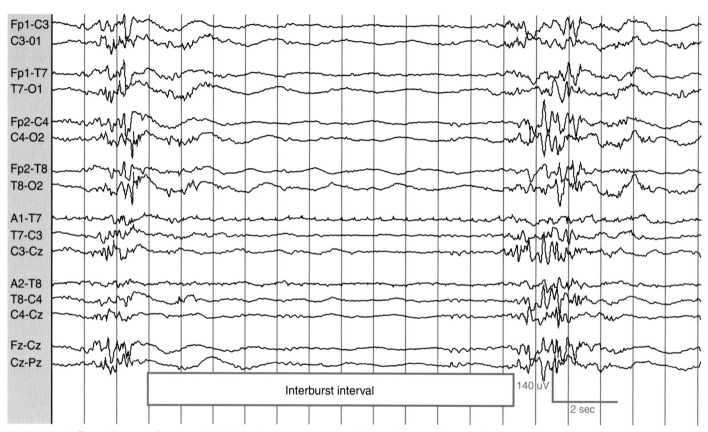

FIGURE 3.1 Tracé discontinu, synchronous. Tracé discontinu pattern seen in a 29.5-week PMA infant. Interburst interval is 9 seconds and bursts are synchronous. Note subtle EKG artifact in A1-T7 channel.

the tracé discontinu is shifting into a less discontinuous pattern called tracé alternant (Fig. 3.2). In tracé alternant, the periods of relative discontinuity are shorter (typically 4–6 seconds) and higher in amplitude (>25 µV). The EEG shows a tracé alternant pattern in quiet sleep and continuous activity in wake and active sleep. Between 37 and 44 weeks PMA, the EEG should be continuous except for quiet sleep, which can maintain a tracé alternant pattern. After 44 weeks, the EEG should be continuous at all times.

Interhemispheric synchrony

The hemispheres are defined as synchronous if there is less than a 1.5 second difference in the onset of EEG activity during a discontinuous background. The development of the neonatal EEG is interesting because synchrony is initially abundant (Fig. 3.1), then decreases, and then increases again. Specifically, premature infants less than 29 weeks have a high level of synchrony (90%–100%). Synchrony nadirs between 31 and 32 weeks PMA, with approximately 50%–70% of bursts being synchronous (Fig. 3.3). After this, synchrony gradually increases (Fig. 3.2). Between 37 and 44 weeks PMA, nearly 100% of bursts (seen during quiet sleep when there is a tracé alternant pattern) are synchronous.

Graphoelements

At different neonatal ages, there is the development of certain characteristic waveforms. These are either not seen in the normal adult EEG (delta brush) or seen in adult life but may have an entirely different significance (sharp waves/transients). The following background elements appear, peak, and then fade during particular periods of neonatal development.

The first characteristic waveform to be seen is the delta brush pattern, which can be present as early as 24 weeks PMA. This is a slow, moderate to high amplitude delta wave with superimposed lower amplitude fast frequencies. Between 24 and 29 weeks PMA, delta brushes are seen mostly over the central and midline areas, but by 32–35 weeks PMA, delta brushes are seen primarily in the occipital and temporal regions (Figs. 3.2, 3.3). Prior to 33 weeks PMA, the delta brushes are seen primarily in active sleep. After 33 weeks PMA, the delta brush pattern is seen primarily in quiet sleep. Delta brushes are infrequent by 37 weeks and if abundant, should be taken as evidence of possible dysmaturity.

Monorhythmic occipital delta activity consists of runs of high amplitude posterior delta. This activity occurs symmetrically and synchronously, usually in the bilateral occipital regions. It has a similar time course as delta brush, first appearing at 24 weeks PMA, peaking between 31 and 33 weeks, and fading by 35 weeks. In an infant less than 29 weeks PMA, monorhythmic occipital delta activity rarely lasts more than a few seconds in duration. By 31 weeks PMA, runs of monorhythmic occipital delta can last for more than 30 seconds, often admixed with delta brush.

Theta bursts, also known as temporal sawtooth waves, are seen starting at 26 weeks PMA and maximal in the relatively narrow PMA bandwidth of between 29 and 32 weeks. These occur in the temporal electrodes independently for 1–2 seconds and consist of sharply contoured rhythmic theta waves, with amplitudes of up to 200 µV.

Starting at 32 weeks, during continuous portions of EEG, there is the development of a rarely present amplitude gradient with higher amplitudes posteriorly (in the delta range) and lower amplitudes, with faster frequency anteriorly. This gradient is maintained in adult life (though the frequencies are different) and becomes the cornerstone of an organized adult EEG.

Multifocal sharp transients (Fig. 3.4) are most frequent between 32 and 34 weeks but can persist and are considered normal up until 46 weeks PMA. These are sharp waves, which can be maximal in essentially any location.

After 34 weeks, frontal sharp waves (also known as encoches frontales) become more frequent as multifocal sharp transients become less frequent.

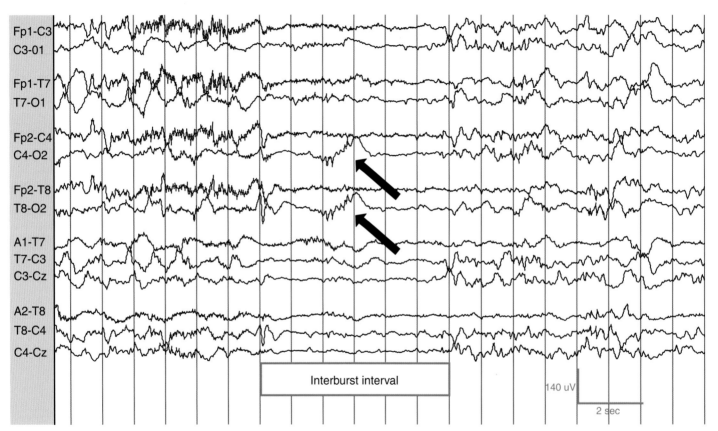

Interburst interval

140 uV

2 sec

FIGURE 3.2 Tracé alternant and delta brush. Tracé alternant pattern seen in quiet sleep in a 35.5-week PMA infant. Interburst interval is 5–6 seconds. Bursts are synchronous. *Arrows* point to right occipital delta brush.

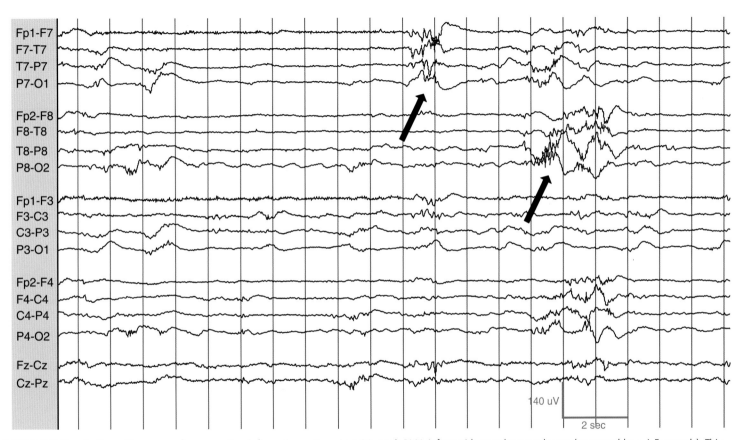

FIGURE 3.3 Tracé discontinu, asynchronous. Tracé discontinu pattern in a 31-week PMA infant with asynchronous bursts (separated by >1.5 seconds). This PMA is the nadir of synchrony. *Arrows* pointed to asynchronous bursts with delta brush.

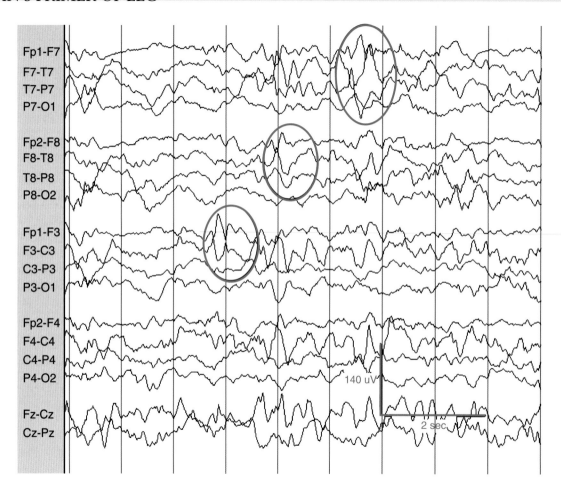

FIGURE 3.4 Multifocal sharp transients.
Multifocal sharp transients seen in this 36-week PMA infant.

Frontal sharp waves usually occur in isolation or in brief runs and are typically synchronous and symmetric (Fig. 3.5). They may appear as early as 26 weeks PMA but are polyphasic, with high amplitudes. They diminish at 44 weeks PMA, are rarely seen during sleep after 46 weeks PMA, and disappear by 48 weeks PMA. Frontal monorhythmic delta is seen around 34 weeks PMA. This pattern often appears with admixed frontal sharp waves. Both multifocal sharp transients and frontal sharp waves can occur in any state. As these have a morphology similar to adult sharp waves, it is a common rookie mistake to report these as abnormal and as markers for a possible seizure disorder. Even if these persist past 46 weeks PMA, they are a more nonspecific sign of cerebral dysfunction and may not be secondary to cortical hyperexcitability. If sharp waves are overly frequent at any one location, occur for long periods of time, and/or have persistent asymmetry, they are abnormal at any age.

Sleep/wake cycle

For the neonate, awake is the behavioral state with the eyes open and asleep is the state with the eyes closed. Before 29 weeks PMA, sleep/wake cycles are not discernible. Respirations are exclusively irregular. Between 29 and 32 weeks PMA, there is the emergence of rarely identifiable quiet and active sleep. At this age, wake and active sleep look the same on the EEG and are continuous. In active sleep, in addition to EEG continuity, there are rapid eye movements (REM), irregular respirations, and increased muscle tone in the submental EMG (chin muscle tone). In quiet sleep, respirations are regular and the EEG shows a tracé discontinu pattern (Fig. 3.6A). Much of sleep remains indeterminate, which means that sleep states cannot be clearly identified as quiet or active sleep.

By 35 weeks PMA, there is a decrease of tonic EMG in active sleep. This is maintained throughout childhood and adult life as muscle tone is low in active sleep/REM sleep. In the pathological circumstance of REM behavior disorder in adults, this paralysis is lost, and people will act out their dreams, resulting in punching, kicking, screaming, leg bicycling, and even getting out of bed. By 35 weeks PMA, a mixed pattern (activité moyenne), which contains both low and medium amplitude components of varying frequencies, dominates the awake and active sleep record (Fig. 3.5). During active sleep at this age, there are more rapid eye movements during REM. Quiet sleep has longer periods of regular respirations.

By 37 weeks PMA, wakefulness, active sleep, and quiet sleep can be clearly delineated on the EEG. Active sleep and wakefulness consist of activité moyenne. At term, approximately 80% of sleep onset and 50% of overall sleep consists of active (REM) sleep. Quiet sleep consists of either a tracé alternant pattern or a continuous slow wave pattern, which is a more mature feature (Fig. 3.6B). In between waking, active sleep, and quiet sleep, there is something called transitional sleep, which represents a behavioral and EEG pattern not completely fulfilling criteria for the above mentioned patterns.

Reactivity

The neonatal EEG is not reactive to stimulation until 32 weeks PMA. After 32 weeks PMA, stimulation will cause either a widespread attenuation of activity or, less often, an augmentation of activity on the EEG. If the baby is in quiet sleep with a tracé alternant pattern, stimulation may cause a transition to a continuous slow pattern. By 41 weeks, occipital lambda waves are sometimes present, with visual fixation.

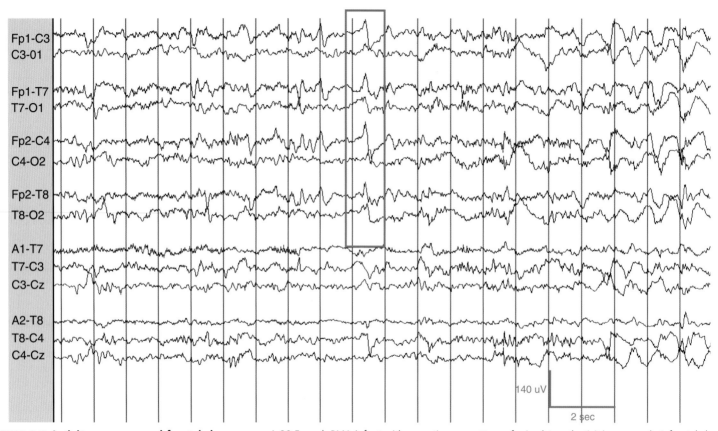

FIGURE 3.5 Activite moyenne and frontal sharp wave. A 39.5-week PMA infant with a continuous pattern of mixed type (activité moyenne). A frontal sharp wave is shown in the *box*.

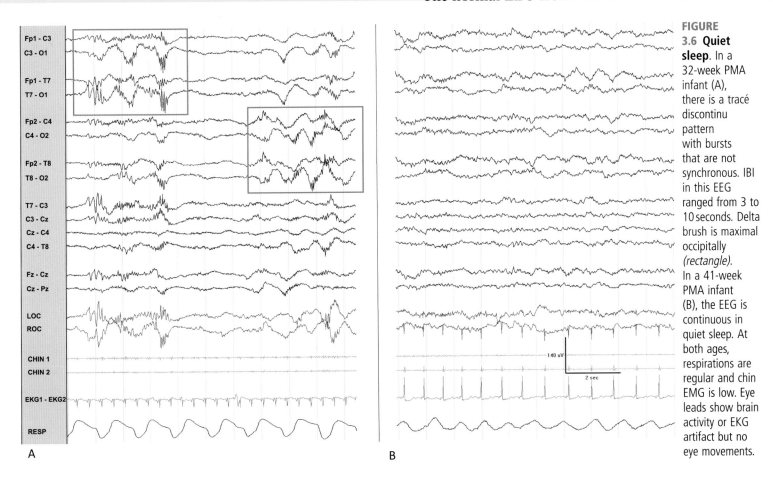

A

B

**FIGURE
3.6 Quiet
sleep**. In a
32-week PMA
infant (A),
there is a tracé
discontinu
pattern
with bursts
that are not
synchronous. IBI
in this EEG
ranged from 3 to
10 seconds. Delta
brush is maximal
occipitally
(rectangle).
In a 41-week
PMA infant
(B), the EEG is
continuous in
quiet sleep. At
both ages,
respirations are
regular and chin
EMG is low. Eye
leads show brain
activity or EKG
artifact but no
eye movements.

EEG FROM FULL TERM TO ADOLESCENCE

In order to understand the EEG in children, we emphasize that variability is the rule—certainly much greater than in adults. The late neonatal features discussed earlier—multifocal sharp waves, tracé alternant, and frontal sharp waves—are rarely seen past 44 weeks PMA.

During the first year of life, there is a gradual shift from delta to theta. Over the next 2 years, delta declines markedly, and at about 3 years, there is predominately diffuse theta with less frequent delta waves. Between ages 3 and 6 years, diffuse theta declines further. By age 8 years, some theta persists, as it does for the next few years. This is where confusion arises. We find a wide range of theta prominence in young subjects, with no demonstrable cerebral pathology on imaging studies and no neurological deficits. Thus unless there is some clinical correlation for "excessive" slowing, particularly in the theta range, it is best to be generous. When in doubt, opt for a declaration of normal rather than abnormal. On the other hand, if there is a great deal of delta after age 4 or 5 years, the odds are that there indeed is cerebral dysfunction. Observe that diffuse slowing, regardless of degree, must be symmetric. Asymmetric slowing is indicative of cerebral dysfunction. Note: It is particularly important to obtain a true waking record in children. They frequently are drowsy, or rapidly become so. Thus assessment of slowing must be made during the alert state.

Awake EEG

The posterior dominant rhythm (PDR) is not present at birth but develops in the majority of infants in the third or fourth month of life and is 3-4 Hz (Fig. 3.7). This rhythm, like its adult counterpart, is present in the wakeful state when the eyes are closed and attenuates with eye opening. At 6 months, for most infants, the PDR is 5 Hz; at 12 months, the PDR is 6 Hz; and at 36 months, the majority of children will have a PDR of 8 Hz (Fig. 3.8). (Hint: It is easier to remember if you start with a PDR of 8 Hz at the age of 3 years and then work backwards—8 Hz, 3 years; 7 Hz, 2 years; 6 Hz, 1 year; 5 Hz, 6 months; 3–4 Hz, 3–4 months). Between 3 years of age and adulthood, the PDR shifts higher in the alpha range (8–13 Hz), and should exceed 8.5 Hz in adults. The amplitude of the PDR is often asymmetric, typically higher in amplitude on the right (the skull on the left is often thicker, conveniently protecting our left-dominant brain). This is normal, as long as the higher amplitude is not greater than two times the lower amplitude.

Features of sleep

In the term infant, the background pattern of quiet sleep transitions from a tracé alternant pattern to a pattern of continuous high-voltage slow activity. In a normal infant, sleep architecture typically begins to develop at 1.5–3 months with the appearance of sleep spindles. These early sleep spindles are several seconds in duration, in a frontocentral location, in the high alpha or low beta range, and are not synchronous (Fig. 3.9). The lack of synchrony is likely due to lack of myelination in the neonatal brain. By 2 years of age, it is considered abnormal if most spindles are still asynchronous (Fig. 3.10). Persistent absence of sleep spindles on one side raises the suspicion for ipsilateral dysfunction. Sleep spindles are part of N2 sleep.

Vertex waves and K-complexes should be well developed by 5–6 months. They can have a similar distribution, both maximal at the vertex of the head. Vertex waves phase reverse, often at the Cz, C3 and/or C4 electrodes in a bipolar montage, and can occur in repetitive runs, particularly in children (Fig. 3.11). Vertex waves have a shorter duration, <200 ms, while K-complexes are often >0.5 seconds. Vertex waves can be seen in N1 and N2 sleep, and K-complexes (like sleep spindles) are part of N2 sleep. K-complexes occur spontaneously and in response to stimulation, particularly noise.

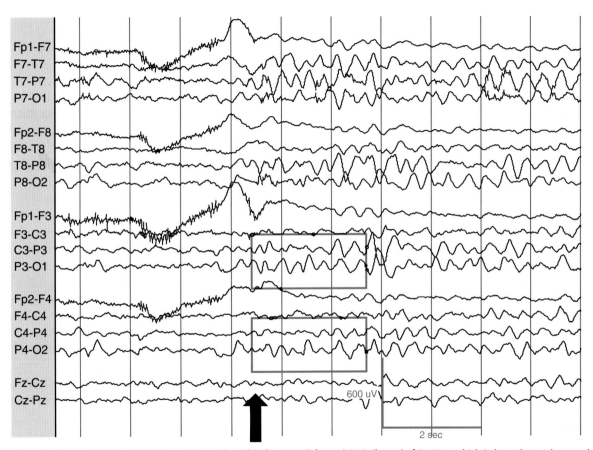

FIGURE 3.7 Posterior dominant rhythm (PDR) in a 4-month-old infant. Well-formed PDR *(boxes)* of 3–4 Hz, which is brought out by eye closure *(arrow)*.

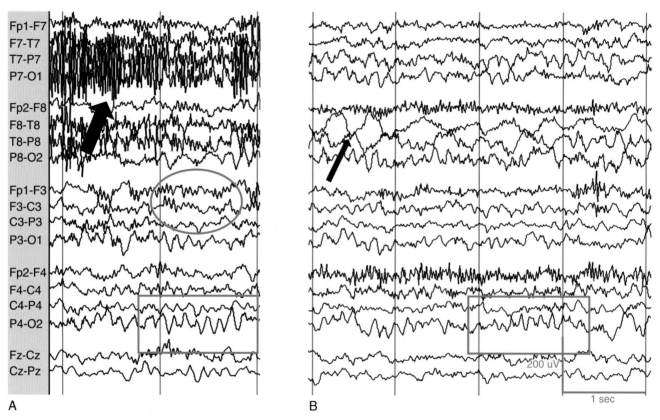

FIGURE 3.8 Posterior dominant rhythm (PDR) in two 2-year-old children. Both (A) and (B) show a well-formed PDR *(boxes)* of 7–8 Hz, with higher amplitude posteriorly and lower amplitude anteriorly. In (A), there is abundant jaw artifact *(thick arrow)*, and low amplitude beta activity is superimposed on theta anteriorly *(oval)*. (B) There is pacifier artifact seen at T8 *(thin arrow)*.

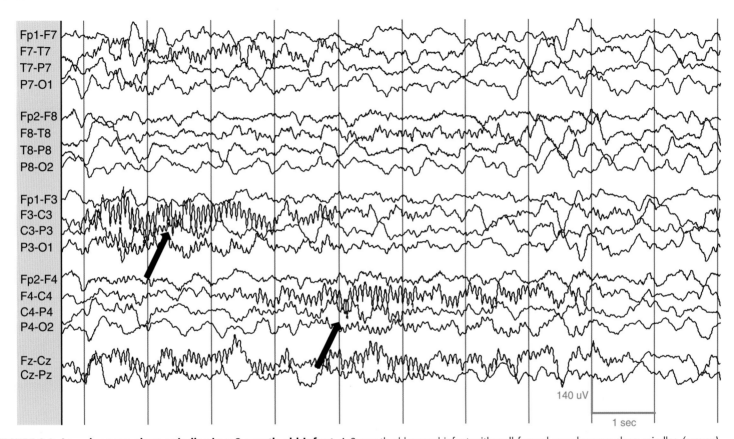

FIGURE 3.9 Asynchronous sleep spindles in a 2-month-old infant. A 2-month-old normal infant with well-formed asynchronous sleep spindles *(arrows)*. Rule of 2: at 2 months of age, sleep spindles appear but are asynchronous. At 2 years of age, sleep spindles become synchronous.

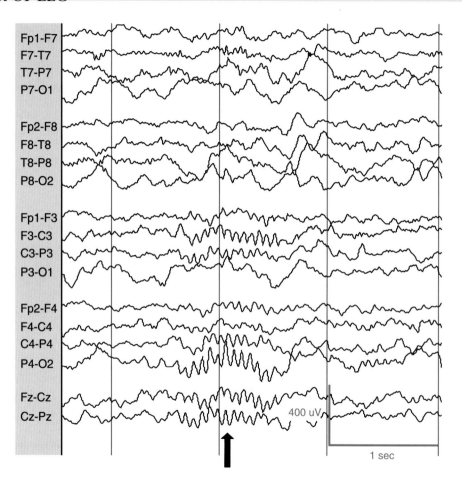

FIGURE 3.10 Synchronous sleep spindles in an 18-month-old infant.

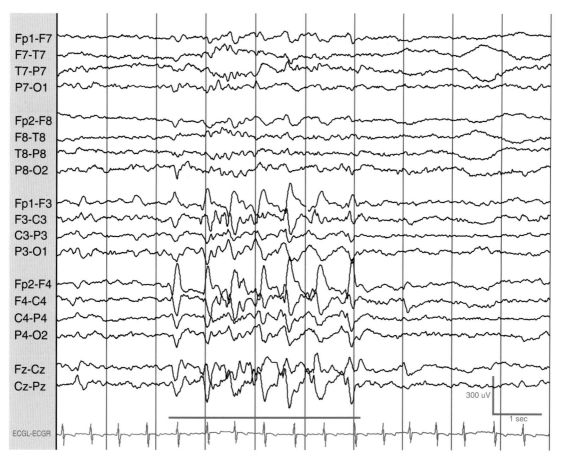

FIGURE 3.11
Vertex waves. A 3-year-old girl with a repetitive run of vertex waves *(line)*.

By 3 months of age, infants typically have a sleep onset consisting of non-REM sleep, which is typical of the normal adult. In addition, REM sleep begins to occupy a lower percentage of total sleep time, going from 50% at full term to 40% at 3 months, and finally, 20% in the adolescent and adult. Within the first year of life, the EEG begins to show sleep stages similar to those of the adult, with N1, N2, N3 (slow wave) and REM sleep.

Normal variants

Half alpha variant

In wake, there are a few normal variants not seen in adults. The half alpha variant can be seen in children, typically after the age of 8. As the name suggests, it is approximately one-half the frequency of the PDR, and often has a notched appearance (Fig. 3.12).

Posterior slow waves of youth

Posterior slow waves of youth occur commonly between 2 and 21 years of age (Fig. 3.13). They are typically in the delta range, consisting of 3–6 fused alpha waves. Both half alpha variant and posterior slow waves of youth should attenuate with eye opening and alerting stimulation.

Hypnogogic/hypnopompic hypersynchrony

In drowsiness, between the ages of 6 months and 2 years, most children will develop a pattern with bursts of diffuse, high voltage (>350 µV) slow waves (3–5 Hz) lasting for several seconds: hypnogogic hypersynchrony. An identical pattern, termed hypnopompic hypersynchrony (Fig. 3.14), can be seen with transitions from sleep to wake. These patterns are rarely seen after adolescence. By approximately age 10, children can have slow roving lateral eye movements in drowsiness. This persists throughout adulthood.

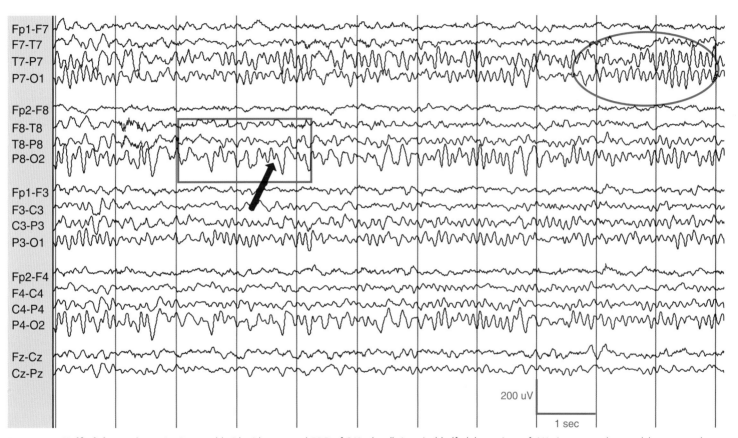

FIGURE 3.12 Half alpha variant. An 8-year-old girl with a normal PDR of 8 Hz *(oval)*. A typical half alpha variant of 4 Hz is present *(rectangle)*, more on the right, with a characteristic notched morphology *(arrow)*.

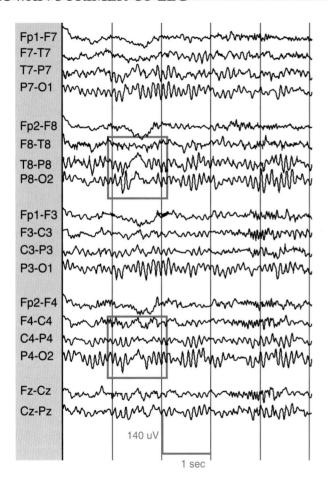

FIGURE 3.13 Posterior slow waves of youth. A 7-year-old boy with a well-formed PDR of 9 Hz with a posterior slow wave of youth seen on the right *(boxes)*.

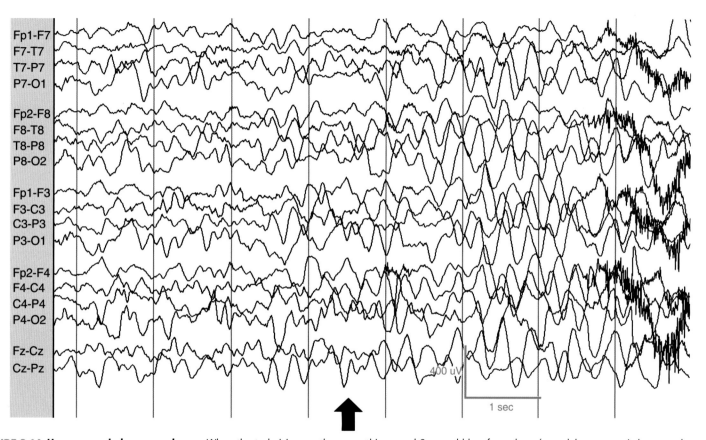

FIGURE 3.14 Hypnopompic hypersynchrony. When the technician gently rouses this normal 2-year-old boy from sleep *(arrow)*, hypnopompic hypersynchrony is seen with high voltage 3 Hz activity.

Table 3.1 Postmenstrual age and the EEG

Postmenstrual age	Continuity	Synchrony	Graphoelements	Sleep/wake cycles	Reactivity
24–29 weeks	**Tracé discontinu:** IBI 6–12 seconds, up to 60 seconds.	90%–100%	**Delta brush:** Located frequently over the central and midline areas. **Monorhythmic occipital delta activity:** Runs last only a few seconds. **Theta bursts:** Appear at 26 weeks.	**No sleep/wake cycles:** Respiration always irregular.	**Not reactive** No state change
29–32 weeks	**Tracé discontinu:** IBI 5–8 seconds, up to 20 seconds. **Continuous activity:** Rare but may be seen in wake and active sleep.	50%–70%	**Delta brush:** More abundant; more prominent in active sleep. **Monorhythmic occipital delta activity:** Runs can last more than 30 seconds. **Theta bursts:** Maximal at this PMA.	**Awake/active sleep:** EEG is continuous. REM seen in active sleep. **Quiet sleep:** Tracé discontinu. **Indeterminate:** Majority of EEG is indeterminate.	**Reactive to stimulation**
32–35 weeks	**Tracé discontinu:** IBI become briefer (<10 seconds). **Continuous activity:** May be seen in wake and active sleep.		**Delta brushes:** Most frequent over temporal and occipital regions. More common in quiet sleep. **Monorhythmic occipital delta activity:** Fading in occipital regions. **Theta bursts:** Cease. **Multifocal sharp transients:** Maximal at this PMA.	**Awake/active sleep:** EEG is continuous. **Quiet sleep:** Tracé discontinu. **Indeterminate:** Much of the EEG is still indeterminate.	**Reactive**

Table 3.1 Postmenstrual age and the EEG—cont'd					
Postmenstrual age	Continuity	Synchrony	Graphoelements	Sleep/wake cycles	Reactivity
35–37 weeks	**Tracé alternant:** Relative discontinuity between 4 and 6 seconds. Seen in quiet sleep. **Continuous activity:** In wake and active sleep.	60%–85%	**Delta brushes:** More frequent during quiet sleep. **Multifocal sharp transients:** Less abundant. **Frontal sharp waves (encoches frontales):** Maximally expressed at this PMA. **Monorhythmic frontal delta**	**Awake:** Activité moyenne pattern dominates. **Active sleep:** REM, decreased EMG, activité moyenne predominates on EEG. **Quiet sleep:** Respirations more regular, tracé alternant pattern on EEG.	**Reactive**
37–44 weeks	**Tracé alternant:** Can be seen in quiet sleep. **Continuous activity:** Majority of record is continuous except quiet sleep, which can show a tracé alternant pattern.	90%–100%	**Delta brushes:** Very infrequent. **Multifocal sharp transients:** Typically resolve. **Frontal sharp waves (encoches frontales):** Diminish by 44 weeks PMA.	**Awake:** Activité moyenne. **Active sleep:** REM, decreased EMG, activité moyenne predominates on EEG. **Quiet sleep:** Respirations more regular, tracé alternant pattern or continuous slow wave pattern.	**Reactive**

IBI, Interburst interval; *PMA,* postmenstrual age; *REM,* rapid eye movement.

Further reading

Battin, M., Rutherford, M., 2001. Magnetic resonance imaging of the brain in preterm infants: 24 weeks' gestation to term. In: Rutherford, M.A. (Ed.), MRI of the Neonatal Brain. WB Saunders, London. (Part 2, Chapter 3)

Blum, W.T., 1982. Atlas of Pediatric EEG. Raven, New York.

Eiserman, M., Kaminska, A., Moutard., 2013. Normal EEG in childhood: From neonates to adolescents. Neurophysiol. Clin 43, 35–65.

Fisch, B.J., 1999. The normal EEG from premature age to the age of 19 years. In: Fisch, B.J. (Ed.), Fisch and Spehlmann's EEG Primer. Elsevier, Oxford, pp. 155–184.

Laoprasert, P., 2011. Atlas of Pediatric EEG. McGraw Hill, London. 201–273.

Marcuse, L.V., Schneider, M., Mortati, K.A., et al., 2008. Quantitative analysis of the EEG posterior-dominant rhythm in healthy adolescents. Clin. Neurophysiol. 119 (8), 1778–1781.

Mizrahi, E., Hrachovy, R., 2015. Atlas of Neonatal Electroencephalography, fourth edition. Demos Medical, New York. 10–123.

St. Louis, E.K., Frey, L.C., 2016. Electroencephalography (EEG): An Introductory Text and Atlas of Normal and Abnormal Findings in Adults, Children, and Infants. American Epilepsy Society, Chicago, IL. 20–39.

Tsuchida, T.N., Wusthoff, C.J., Shelhass, R.A., et al., 2013. American Clinical Neurophysiology Society standardized EEG terminology and categorization for the description of continuous EEG monitoring in neonates: report of the American Clinical Neurophysiology Society Critical Care Monitoring Committee. J. Clin. Neurophysiol. 30 (2),161–173.

Valentine, D., 2020. https://www.learningeeg.com/neonatal.

Westmoreland, B.F., Klass, D.W., 1996. Electroencephalography: Electroencephalograms of neonates, infants and children. In: Daube, J. (Ed.), Clinical Neurophysiology. FA Davis, Philadelphia, pp. 104–113.

BACKGROUND ABNORMALITIES

Organization

In the awake state, in a well-organized EEG, there is a well-formed posterior dominant rhythm (PDR) occipitally, which attenuates with eye opening. Anteriorly, the frequencies are faster and lower in amplitude. This is referred to as the normal anterior-posterior (A-P) gradient. In sleep, there are distinct sleep states with sleep structures (e.g., K-complexes, vertex waves) specific to each state. If these elements are entirely lacking, the EEG is said to be poorly organized. If an individual has some elements of normal organization but not all, the organization is described as fair.

Diffuse slowing

The presence of diffuse slowing suggests bilateral cerebral dysfunction with a broad spectrum of causes. The first major problem in making a determination of diffuse slowing is the patient's state of alertness. Many patients are quite drowsy throughout a routine EEG recording. This, of course, produces slowing of the record that would not necessarily be abnormal. The electroencephalographer must diagnose the presence of diffuse slowing during the most alert segments of recording. If this is not possible, one may have to say that the diffuse slowing may be in part, if not wholly, due to drowsiness, although a degree of cerebral pathology cannot be excluded. For patients with a depressed level of consciousness, the degree of slowing is determined after an alerting stimuli (often nail bed pressure) (Fig. 4.1).

When an alert segment is encountered, the PDR, if present, is determined. In adults, a PDR <8.5 Hz is abnormal. If the abnormal PDR is symmetric, this is usually not secondary to a focal (e.g., posterior) problem, but a diffuse abnormality. In addition, abundant theta in the awake adult record or abundant delta in the awake child record usually indicates diffuse slowing, which correlates with either diffuse or multifocal cerebral dysfunction.

In adults, mild slowing is used if the primary background frequency is in the high theta range (7–8 Hz), moderate slowing is used if the frequencies are mainly in the mid theta range (4–7 Hz), and severe slowing is used if the frequencies are mainly in the delta range (0–<4 Hz). Of note, diffuse slowing does not always correlate with the degree of cerebral dysfunction. The classic example of this is in alpha coma where there is no slowing, but there is severe cerebral dysfunction.

A second problem relates to medication. We encounter this frequently, especially with referrals from psychiatry. Many psychotropic drugs (e.g., phenothiazines, lithium, and clozapine) can cause diffuse slowing. While it is true that the record is abnormal in such cases, the patient may demonstrate no obvious neurological dysfunction. Thus when reporting this abnormality, it is important to state that the background slowing may be due to an effect of medication(s) that the patient is taking. Many pathologic processes, including degenerative diseases, congenital structural abnormalities, and toxic metabolic states, can lead to diffuse slowing, as well as slowing of the PDR.

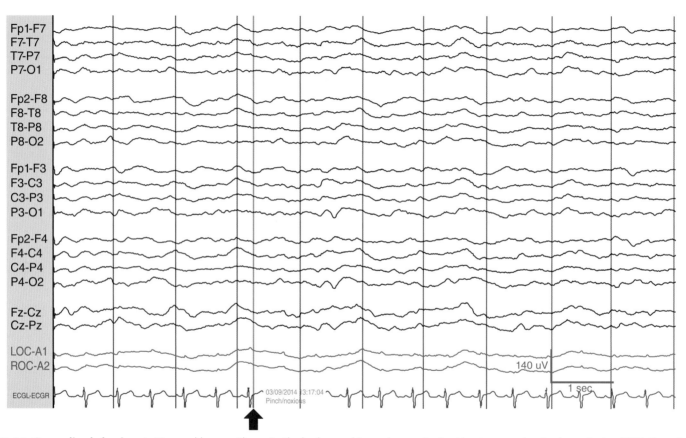

FIGURE 4.1 Generalized slowing. A 46-year-old man with sepsis. The background is poorly organized, without a posterior dominant rhythm (PDR). There is generalized background slowing, consisting mainly of delta frequencies. There is no EEG reactivity to noxious stimulus *(arrow)*.

Focal slowing

As we have seen, slow waves in and of themselves are not abnormal, but slowing that is localized or lateralized commands our attention. In fact, the EEG is highly sensitive to the presence of localized cerebral pathology, often more so than imaging studies. The most important focal abnormality is delta activity (0–<4 Hz) occurring in any cerebral location. Focal delta waves are a good indicator of structural disease. At times, focal delta may not correlate with an evident structural lesion on MRI/CT studies, even though cerebral pathology of some degree underlies the EEG finding (e.g., frontotemporal slowing in nonlesional temporal lobe epilepsy).

Structural lesions producing focal delta include brain tumors, cerebral infarctions, brain abscesses, subdural hematomas, intracerebral hemorrhages, and other traumatic brain injuries. Focal rhythmic (monomorphic) and polymorphic delta activity can be present interictally in patients with focal seizures, with or without clear structural lesions. Delta foci are often most evident in the temporal derivations, even when the main pathology is not in the temporal lobe. We term this false localization, the slowing being projected to the temporal regions from deeper or adjacent structures.

Polymorphic delta is thought to be generated from lesions involving the white matter (Fig. 4.2). Contrast this with rhythmic delta activity that can result from lesions of gray matter—usually cortical. Polymorphic and rhythmic delta often coexist when lesions involve both cortex and subcortical white matter.

Focal attenuation

Fast activity is believed to be generated at the level of the cerebral cortex, so focal attenuation of fast activity is a useful marker of abnormal cortical function. It can happen in acute cortical injury, such as ischemic stroke. It can also occur in the setting of an intervening fluid collection between the scalp and the brain, such as a subdural hematoma (Fig. 4.3).

Breach rhythm

The breach rhythm results from an area of skull defect, usually a post-surgical finding. In the case of a breach artifact, the waveforms are often sharply contoured at higher amplitudes. The technicians are asked to note the presence of craniotomy scars in order to correctly identify this rhythm. Due to the prior surgery, breach rhythms are often associated with focal slowing (Fig. 4.4).

Continuity

The normal EEG should be continuous. As the brain becomes more dysfunctional, it becomes less organized and slower and can have periods of diffuse attenuation ($\geq$10 µV but <50% of background voltage) or suppression (<10 µV). When the periods of attenuation or suppression consist of 10%–49% percent of the recording, the background is called "discontinuous." If these periods exceed 50% of the recording, the background is in a "burst-suppression pattern" (Fig. 4.5). The "bursts" should last $\geq$0.5 seconds; otherwise, the bursts are considered "discharges" occurring out of suppressed or attenuated background. The burst-suppression pattern can be medically induced, for example, in patients in status epilepticus, or can be present without any sedating medications, such as in cardiac arrest patients.

Reactivity and state changes

Having a PDR automatically means that the EEG is reactive. When a brain is more dysfunctional, the PDR disappears and often, normal sleep transients are absent. There can still be rudimentary sleep-wake cycles in the EEG background, consistent with state change. To be considered a state change, it must last for >60 seconds and be reproducible with alerting stimulation. For example, in a more awake state, whether by spontaneous arousal or by stimulation, the EEG may become more

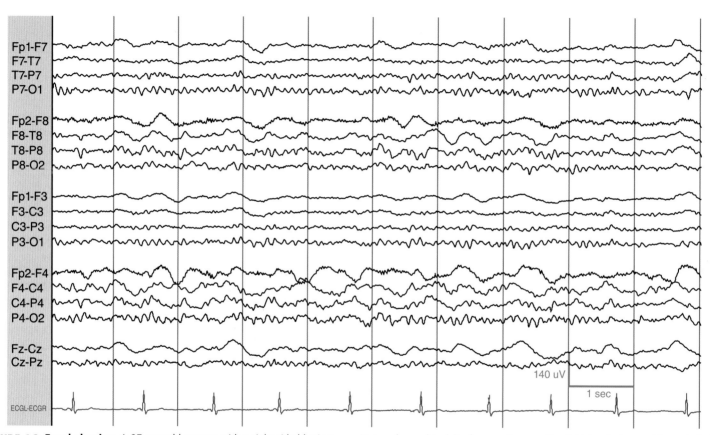

FIGURE 4.2 Focal slowing. A 27-year-old woman with a right-sided brain tumor. Note polymorphic delta frequencies over the right hemisphere, with a relatively preserved posterior dominant rhythm.

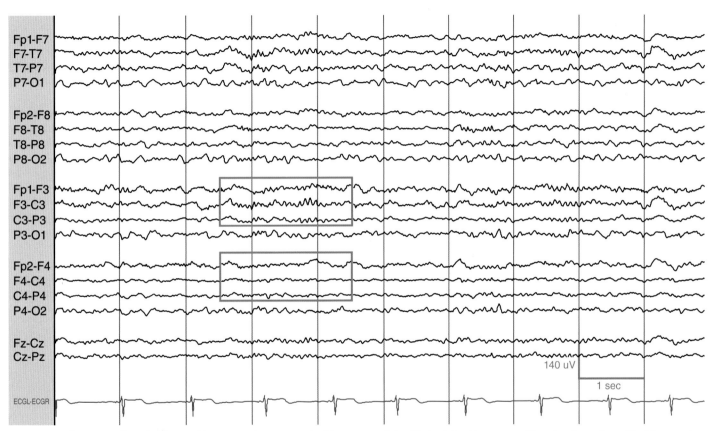

FIGURE 4.3 Focal attenuation. A 66-year-old woman who presented with an acute right-sided subdural hematoma. There is attenuation of fast frequencies over the right side compared with the left side *(boxes)*.

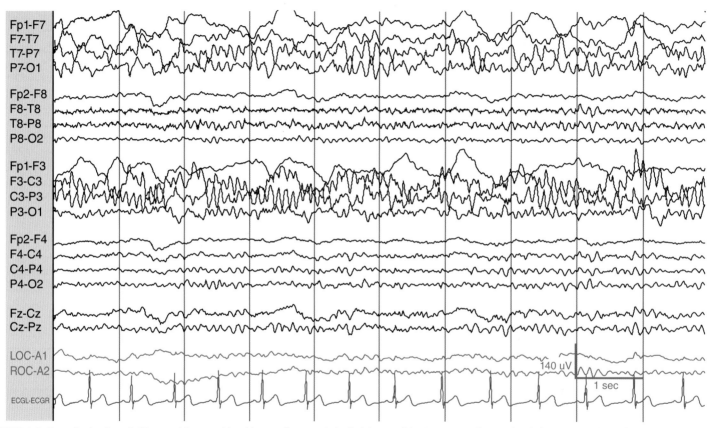

FIGURE 4.4 Breach rhythm. A 21-year-old man with a history of traumatic brain injury and brain surgery. There is focal slowing over the left hemisphere, and a breach rhythm is seen most prominently over the left frontoparietal region.

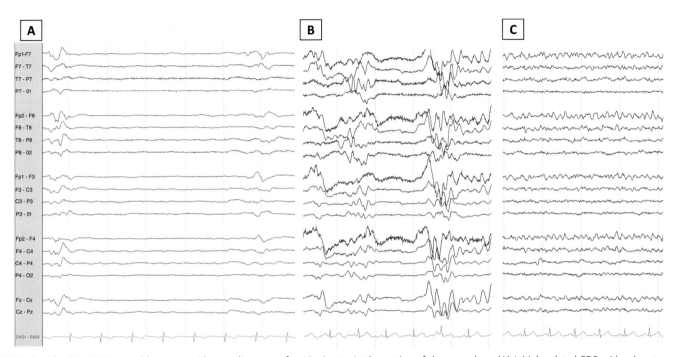

FIGURE 4.5 Continuity. A 56-year-old women with a cardiac arrest for 10 minutes in the setting of drug overdose. (A) Initial sedated EEG with a burst-suppression pattern, with >50% of the record suppressed (<10 µV). (B) As sedation is weaned, the EEG is discontinuous, with 10%–49% of the record attenuated or suppressed. (C) Off sedation, the EEG is continuous but disorganized.

continuous, with faster frequencies. The presence of state change means that there is reactivity.

With worsened cerebral function, state changes can be lost. However, there still can be reactivity, which means that there is a <60 second change in cerebral EEG activity in response to stimulation. This change is usually an increase in frequency of cerebral rhythms, but diffuse attenuation is a version of reactivity. It is important to note that eye blinks or muscle artifact do not signify EEG reactivity. The absence of EEG reactivity is a generally poor prognostic sign in the absence of sedating medications.

Stimulation-induced rhythmic, periodic, or ictal-appearing discharges (SIRPIDs) are a pathological response to stimulation often seen in critically ill patients.

EPILEPTIFORM DISCHARGES, PERIODIC OR RHYTHMIC PATTERNS

Epileptiform discharges

In patients with epilepsy, despite the important role of the EEG, the diagnosis often rests on clinical grounds. Rarely, epileptiform discharges can be recorded in persons without epilepsy. Likewise, patients with epilepsy can have a normal EEG between seizures. Nonetheless, the EEG provides important supporting evidence for a diagnosis of epilepsy. Moreover, the type of epilepsy may be confirmed or even diagnosed. For example, the EEG differentiates between focal and generalized epilepsies and is a principal feature in the definition of epilepsy syndromes.

The following paragraphs provide direction concerning specific findings in epilepsy.

The spike, the spike-wave complex, and polyspikes

The spike is defined as a paroxysmal potential (i.e., it arises suddenly from the background) that is very sharp in contour (you can prick your finger on it) and whose rise usually has a steeper slope than that of its decline. Its duration is 20–70 ms, thus differentiating it from more rapid muscle action potentials. Spikes are usually electronegative at the surface, although there are exceptions. The spike is usually followed by a low-voltage slow potential (duration of about 200 ms) before the baseline is reestablished. In some cases, the slow wave may not be evident. Spikes

may occur in isolation, in groups of two or more, or in repetitive runs (Fig. 4.6). They may be focal, multifocal, or generalized.

The spike-wave complex consists of two components—the spike and the accompanying time-locked slow wave. The prototype is the generalized spike-wave complex recorded in patients with absence epilepsy (Fig. 4.7). In this case, the complex is in the 3 Hz frequency band. The discharge is relatively high in voltage (say 200–300 µV or more) and the slow wave is often higher in amplitude than the spike. A polyspike-wave is a series of spikes occurring before the slow wave (Fig. 4.8). Another distinctive pattern is the generalized irregular polyspike-wave discharge at 4–6 Hz, characteristic of juvenile myoclonic epilepsy (JME).

Spike-wave complexes also occur at frequencies other than 3 Hz. The prototype of slow spike-wave (1.5–2.5 Hz) occurs in Lennox–Gastaut syndrome (LGS) and is generalized at times, with a bifrontal preponderance.

The sharp wave

The sharp wave is defined as a paroxysmal sharp potential (not as pointed as a spike) that has a duration of 70–200 ms (Fig. 4.9). The duration cutoff between spikes and sharp waves is somewhat arbitrary, and the clinical significance is not so different; however, certain epilepsy syndromes have characteristic epileptiform potentials. A sharp wave is typically followed by a slow wave.

Other interictal paroxysmal waveforms

Patients with long-standing epilepsy and generalized seizures, possibly in remission, commonly have generalized irregular slow-wave discharges, sometimes with sharp components. Patients with absence epilepsy may demonstrate brief rhythmic high-voltage 3 Hz slow-wave discharges without accompanying spikes. Such discharges probably represent a forme fruste of 3 Hz spike-wave activity.

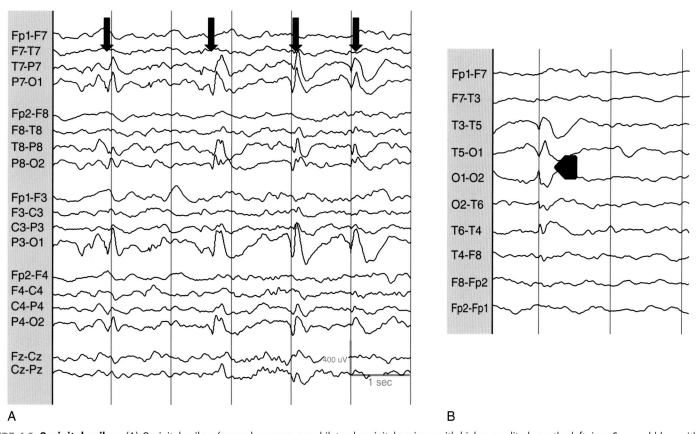

A

B

FIGURE 4.6 Occipital spikes. (A) Occipital spikes *(arrows)* are seen over bilateral occipital regions, with higher amplitude on the left, in a 6-year-old boy with childhood occipital visual epilepsy (COVE). (B) In the circumferential montage, a phase reversal at O1 is seen *(arrowhead)*.

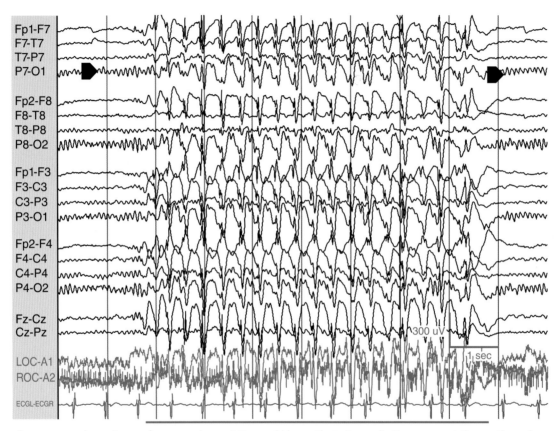

FIGURE 4.7 Spike and wave complexes in an absence seizure. A 7-year-old boy with staring spells. You can count three spike and wave complexes per second (3 Hz spike and wave) *(line)*. Before and after the spike-wave complexes, a clear posterior dominant rhythm (PDR) of 11 Hz can be appreciated *(arrowhead)*.

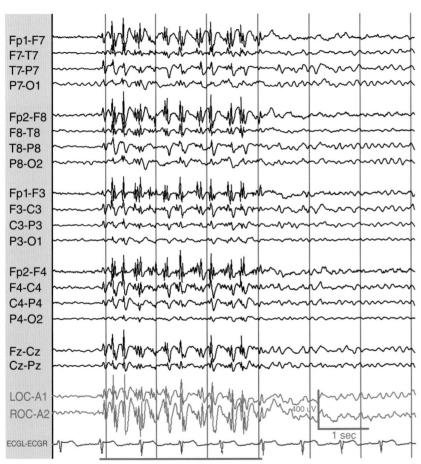

FIGURE 4.8 Polyspike and wave. A 9-year-old girl with generalized tonic-clonic seizures with 3–4 Hz generalized polyspike and wave for 3 seconds (line).

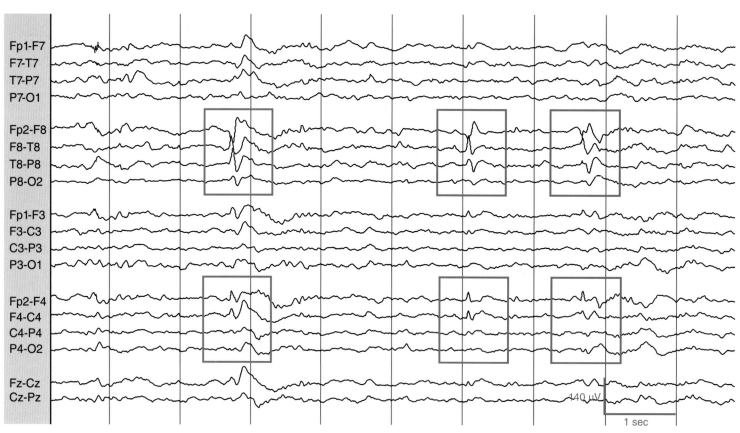

FIGURE 4.9 Frontotemporal sharp waves. Right frontotemporal sharp waves *(boxes)*, with maximum negativity (phase reversing) at F8, are seen in a 33-year-old woman with right mesial temporal sclerosis.

Location and significance of focal epileptiform discharges

Temporal epileptiform discharges

The most common sites for focal epileptiform activity are the temporal lobes. In patients with temporal lobe epilepsy, the discharges may be maximal in the anterior temporal regions (F7/F8 electrodes) (Fig. 4.9). Of note, the F7/F8 electrodes also record spikes originating from the inferior frontal cortex. The temporal lobe discharges may demonstrate a focal maximum between the anterior and midtemporal electrodes (F7/T7 or F8/T8), or indeed, at the midtemporal electrodes (T7/T8). Some laboratories employ F9 and F10 electrodes placed inferior to F7/F8. The temporal lobe spike may be more evident and of higher amplitude at these locations.

The majority of patients with temporal lobe epilepsy will have interictal epileptiform discharges. The frequency of recorded discharges, however, has a weak correlation with the patient's seizure control, although it is true that the number of discharges tends to decline in persistently seizure-free patients.

If epileptiform discharges are present bilaterally in the temporal lobes, it is difficult to determine, on grounds of the EEG, which temporal lobe generates the clinical seizure activity. The more active focus may not be responsible for the patient's recurrent seizures, as has been shown with intensive video-EEG monitoring. Alternatively, the seizures may emanate from either temporal lobe at various times.

Midtemporal epileptiform discharges may have a different significance than discharges that are more anterior. Such discharges may be seen after significant head trauma or with a temporal lobe tumor, resulting in damage to the temporal cortex.

Note that posterior temporal/parietal epileptiform discharges (P7/P8) usually result from more posterior temporal cortical damage and may result from infarction or other pathology in the region of the posterior cerebral circulation.

Occipital epileptiform discharges

The occipital epileptiform discharge focus (O1/O2) is distinctive and usually found in children with occipital epilepsy (see Table 5.2, Epilepsy syndromes and other epilepsies). Care must be taken in discovering its existence for it is easy to concentrate on other brain areas, particularly the temporal regions, and neglect the occipital regions save for determining the frequency of the PDR. This is especially true when the spikes are infrequent for they are easily obscured by ongoing background activity. Important to note is the downward deviation of the epileptiform discharges in the occipital channels in the longitudinal bipolar montage. There is no phase reversal because the occipital electrode is the last in the chain.

An electrode arrangement (montage) that is useful in recording occipital events is referred to as the circumferential montage. Here the electrodes are linked around the scalp, running through the occipital and frontopolar regions. Thus any occipital spike will demonstrate a phase reversal at O1 or O2 (Fig. 4.6). A referential montage can be useful as well and will simply demonstrate the highest amplitude at the occipital electrode. Note also that occipital epileptiform discharges may manifest in both occipital regions, the side of higher amplitude being the putative focus.

The clinical history may help in directing attention to the occipital regions inasmuch as such patients may report visual symptoms consisting of bright or flashing lights or a grid pattern (not formed visual hallucinations such as scenes or persons). Formed visual hallucinations (e.g., "I see my grandmother wearing that floral apron") usually occur in patients with focal seizures of temporal neocortical origin. The EEG diagnosis is important in that occipital epilepsy presenting in childhood usually has a favorable prognosis, both for immediate seizure control and eventual seizure subsidence. The same may not apply to adults.

Centrotemporal epileptiform discharges

Centrotemporal epileptiform discharges are distinctive and, once seen, are not forgotten. They are the accompaniment of self-limited epilepsy with centrotemporal spikes (SeLECTS, formerly known as childhood epilepsy with centrotemporal spikes or benign rolandic epilepsy). The discharges are clearly focal, with maximum negativity (i.e., phase reversal) at the centrotemporal area (C3/T7, C4/T8). Alternatively, the discharges may be maximal in the central and parietal areas (C3/P3, C4/P4), and occipital spikes may coexist. Characteristically, there is a horizontal dipole: negative maxima in the centrotemporal electrodes and positive maxima in the frontal area (Fig. 4.10). They are best seen in the average referential montage. It means that the spike generator is located tangential to the surface electrode as opposed to perpendicular (like most other spike discharges).

Frontal and frontopolar epileptiform discharges

These discharges can be recorded in patients with seizures originating in either frontal lobe or with generalized seizures. The frontopolar epileptiform discharge (Fp1/Fp2) is thought to be generated by orbital frontal cortex or adjacent areas, whereas the frontal epileptiform discharge at the midfrontal electrode(s) (F3/F4) is generated by the frontal convexity. For example, a right frontopolar spike when recorded on a longitudinal bipolar montage is an upgoing potential in channels Fp2/F8 and Fp2/F4. As in the case of occipital spikes, there is no phase reversal (Fp1/2 are the first electrodes in the chain) in a standard montage. These discharges are well displayed with the circumferential montage (Fig. 4.11). As with occipital spikes, there is often representation in the opposite hemisphere at lower voltage. In addition, a focal frontal epilepsy may have interictal discharges that are bilaterally synchronous, with equal amplitude on both sides. In addition, an individual with generalized epilepsy may have spike fragments that are lateralized and frontally predominant. To make matters more confusing, a right mesial frontal focus may create a spike on the EEG that phase reverses on the left, say at the F3 electrode. This is because the synchronous excitatory post synaptic potentials (EPSPs) responsible for any epileptiform discharge create a negative charge along the cortical surface. When that cortical surface is in the mesial right frontal lobe, the negative dipole may project best onto the left frontocentral area, simply because of geometry. When this occurs, it is called false lateralization.

Midline epileptiform discharges

We often say that during drowsiness or sleep, any sharp potential discharge occurring at one of the midline electrodes should be regarded as a normal phenomenon (vertex sharp waves) unless proven otherwise. However, epilepsy foci on the mesial surface of the cerebral hemispheres can cause interictal discharges which are maximal at midline electrodes (Fz, Cz, or Pz). Distinguishing between an epileptiform abnormality and a vertex wave can be difficult. If midline spikes are seen in wakefulness, they are definitely abnormal.

Rhythmic patterns

These patterns can be seen in patients with epilepsy, but they are more commonly seen in patients who are critically ill. Nowadays, continuous EEG monitoring is more widely used to assess brain function in critically ill patients, and these patterns are frequently encountered. In order to facilitate communication and aid in further research, the American Clinical Neurophysiology Society (ACNS) has published and revised the standardized ICU EEG nomenclature, which is used in the following discussions (Table 4.1). Here we will focus on generalized and lateralized rhythmic and periodic patterns.

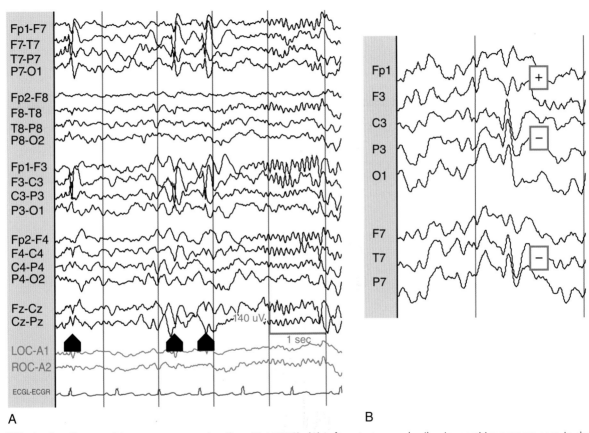

FIGURE 4.10 Self-limited epilepsy with centrotemporal spikes (SeLECTS). (A) Left centrotemporal spikes in repetitive runs are seen in sleep (note spindles) in an 8-year-old boy. (B) A left-sided centrotemporal spike in an average montage. Fp1 and F3 are electropositive (downward deflection), and C3, P3, and T7 are electronegative (upward deflection) on the average montage. This is the horizontal dipole.

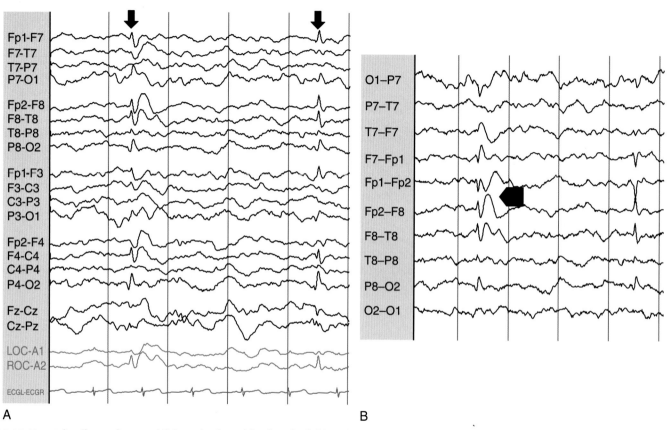

FIGURE 4.11 Frontal spike and wave. (A) Frontal spikes with a broader field on the right are seen in a 5-year-old girl. (B) On the circumferential montage *(right side)*, phase reversal at Fp2 is seen.

Generalized rhythmic delta activity (GRDA)

The term GRDA is used to describe repetitive waveforms that are monomorphic, at least 6 cycles in duration, and rhythmic (think of a very smooth ride on your scooter) in the delta frequency. Frontally predominant GRDA (Fig. 4.12) is most typically seen in adults, whereas occipitally predominant GRDA is more commonly seen in children. The occipitally predominant GRDA is often seen in children with absence epilepsy. Frontally predominant GRDA is a more nonspecific pattern and can be indicative of a toxic-metabolic encephalopathy, a process that involves deep midline structures, subcortical or cortical structural lesions, and/ or raised intracranial pressure. It must be differentiated from repetitive eye blink artifact (Fig. 1.18). A differential point is posterior extension of the potential field in the case of frontally predominant GRDA, while eye blink artifact is usually confined to the frontal regions. Most laboratories employ two periorbital electrodes, one on the lateral lower aspect of the left canthus and the other on the lateral upper aspect of the right canthus. During eye blinks, these eye leads will be mirror images of each other, while during frontally predominant GRDA, the eye leads will be synchronous and symmetric.

Lateralized rhythmic delta activity (LRDA)

When the RDA lateralizes to one side of the brain, it is termed LRDA. LRDA can be present in any particular lobe (frontal, parietal, temporal, occipital), or may appear broadly in one hemisphere (Fig. 4.13). According to the ACNS critical care EEG terminology, if there is bilateral synchronous RDA with a clear predominance of one hemisphere, it is termed LRDA, bilateral asymmetric. LRDA is most often seen when there is a lesion in the gray matter and is often associated with focal cortical hyperexcitability and a tendency toward seizures from that location.

Periodic patterns

This EEG term refers to a periodic pattern consisting of discharges occurring at more or less fixed intervals. Periodic discharges are indicative of significant cerebral disease, whether focal or generalized.

Generalized periodic discharges (GPDs)

These are generalized, synchronous discharges that recur at a certain interval. The discharges vary in waveform but are usually characterized by synchronous high-voltage spikes or sharp waves. GPDs are usually accompanied by a severely abnormal background because of some underlying process that is causing severe bihemispheric dysfunction (Fig. 4.14). In general, GPDs can be seen in a diverse array of clinical conditions, including hypoxic-ischemic encephalopathy, severe toxic-metabolic encephalopathy, Creutzfeldt–Jakob disease (CJD), or subacute sclerosing panencephalitis (SSPE), which is caused by the measles virus (rare now, thanks to vaccination). GPDs, particularly in a toxic-metabolic encephalopathy, may have a triphasic morphology and can have an anterior to posterior lag. GPDs are also often seen in relation to intermittent seizures and convulsive or nonconvulsive status epilepticus (see Chapter 7).

Lateralized periodic discharges (LPDs)

LPDs are repetitive discharges that occur at regular intervals, maximally involving one hemisphere. The discharges may not be epileptiform and may consist, for example, of blunt sharply contoured delta waves that occur periodically. LPDs are most commonly associated with an acute structural lesion involving the cortex. Therefore other findings of focal dysfunction such as focal slowing or attenuation are frequently accompanied in the ipsilateral hemisphere (Fig. 4.15). The most common etiology

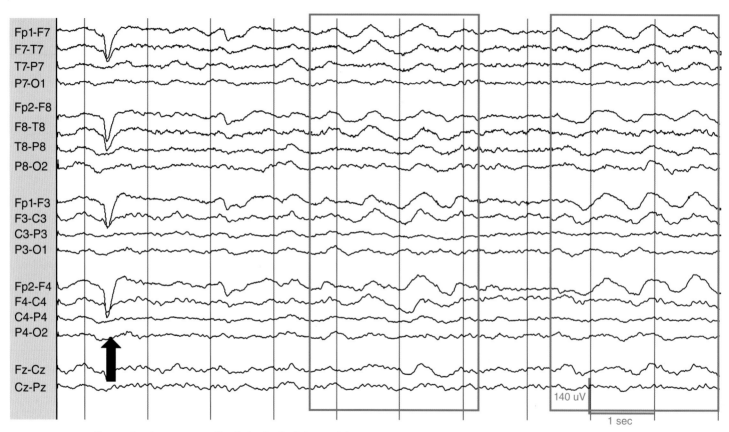

FIGURE 4.12 Frontally predominant generalized rhythmic delta activity (GRDA). A 32-year-old man who developed fever and altered mental status after a small bowel resection. After an eye blink artifact *(arrow)*, frontally predominant GRDA at 1 Hz is shown *(boxes)*.

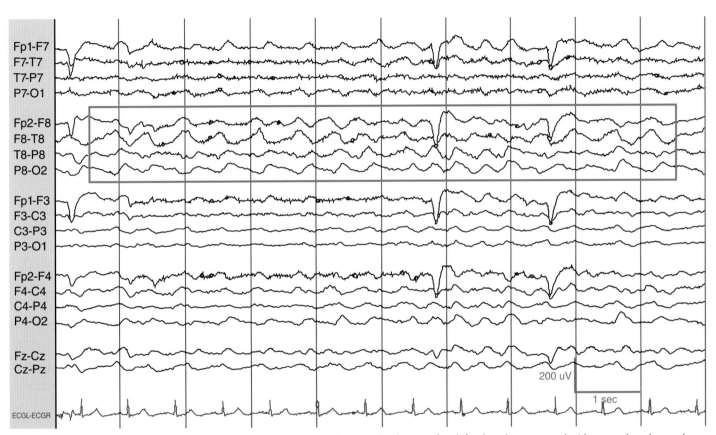

FIGURE 4.13 Lateralized rhythmic delta activity (LRDA). A 63-year-old man with a history of multifocal strokes presented with acute altered mental status. Rhythmic delta activity is seen over the right hemisphere, most prominently over the temporal chain.

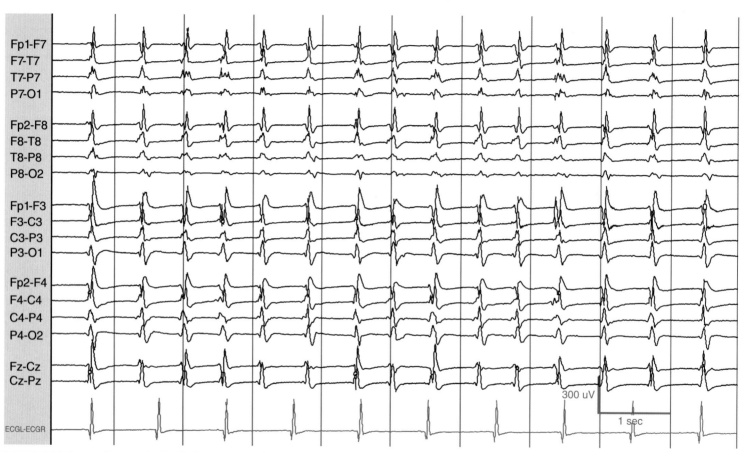

FIGURE 4.14 Generalized periodic discharges (GPDs). 1–2 Hz generalized periodic spike/sharp waves in this 45-year-old woman intubated for status epilepticus.

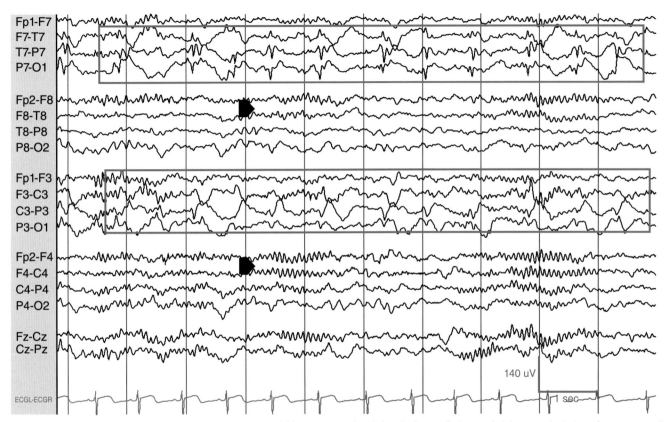

FIGURE 4.15 Lateralized periodic discharges (LPDs). A 9-year-old boy presented with headache, confusion, and right gaze deviation after an appendectomy. He was found to have a left transverse sinus venous thrombosis. EEG shows posteriorly predominant left hemisphere slowing and periodic spike waves occurring at 1 Hz *(boxes)*. Additionally, notice that sleep spindles are seen better on the right *(arrowhead)*.

of LPDs is ischemic stroke. Other frequent etiologies include viral encephalitis (particularly associated with but not limited to herpes simplex virus, with frequent involvement of the temporal lobe), brain tumors, brain abscesses, and intracranial hemorrhages. LPDs may be seen without any obvious structural lesion. It is common to see LPDs in a location adjacent to the acute injury, presumably due to the relative inactivity of the severely damaged cortex. Bilateral independent PDs that are not synchronous are often caused by bilateral structural lesions (Fig. 4.17).

Sometimes it is difficult to determine whether LPDs represent an ictal pattern or not, thus whether to treat LPDs or not. In epilepsia partialis continua, focal clonic seizures can occur in a time-locked pattern to the contralateral LPDs. This clearly represents ongoing seizures. If the LPDs are greater than 2.5 Hz for ≥10 seconds or if there is electrographic evolution lasting ≥10 seconds, the pattern is considered ictal on electrographic criteria alone. Evolution is defined as at least two unequivocal, sequential changes in frequency, morphology, or location. However, we may encounter situations that are not so clear, which is called "the ictal-interictal continuum (Fig. 7.10)." When there is no definite clinical motor manifestation, look for other signs such as eye deviation, nystagmus, hemiparesis, sensory disturbances, aphasia, hemianopsia, or a depressed level of consciousness. In these cases, treatment with antiseizure medications (ASMs) should be considered, especially if there is not a structural lesion that clearly explains the neurological deficits. If clinical improvement along with improvement of LPDs is seen with a benzodiazepine or a loading dose of a fast-acting ASM, it suggests that the pattern was ictal, and in this case, further ASM management is indicated.

Further terms and modifiers of rhythmic and periodic patterns

According to current ACNS nomenclature, additional features which render more ictal-appearing patterns are described with plus (+) modifiers (Table 4.1). For PDs, the modifiers include superimposed fast activity (F) (Fig. 4.17), rhythmic activity (R) (Fig. 4.18), or both (FR). For RDA, the modifiers include superimposed fast activity (F) or spike/sharp waves (S) (Fig. 4.19), or both (FS). Patterns of RDA+ and PD+ are considered to have a higher association with seizures than RDA or PD alone. The plus modifiers do not apply to the term SW, which connotes a pattern of spike and wave or sharp and wave, and is used in patterns of spike/sharp and wave where there is no interval between one spike-wave complex and the next (Fig. 4.20).

Of note, rhythmic and periodic patterns or even seizures can become activated with various stimuli (from clinical examinations, nursing care, noxious stimuli, environmental sounds, spontaneous arousal, etc.), and these phenomena are described as stimulus-induced rhythmic, periodic, or ictal discharges (SIRPIDs) (Fig. 4.21).

Brief potentially ictal rhythmic discharges (BIRDs)

BIRDs are very brief (≥0.5 to <10 seconds) runs of focal or generalized rhythmic activity >4 Hz with or without evolution, not consistent with a known normal pattern or benign variant. In addition, they cannot be part of a burst-suppression or burst attenuation pattern. The nonevolving BIRDs typically last for 0.5–4 seconds (Fig. 4.22). Seen in both critically ill and non-critically ill patients, they are associated with high risk of seizures and are highly correlated with the seizure focus. These discharges can display rapid bisynchrony and appear generalized, even when a focal source is known. The term paroxysmal fast activity (PFA), which could be considered as a subtype of BIRDs, has similar clinical significance, whether it is generalized (GPFA) or focal. (Fig. 4.23). Close correlation with clinical behavior is warranted, especially with GPFA, as tonic seizures can be very subtle clinically, in which case, it would be a seizure. This is common in patients with LGS during sleep.

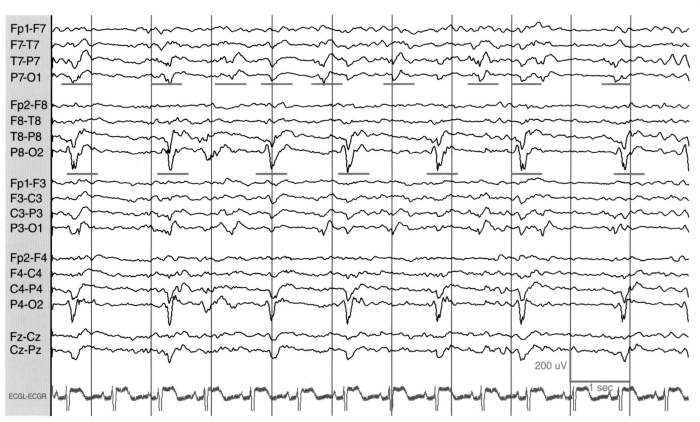

FIGURE 4.16 Bilateral independent periodic discharges (BIPDs). A 64-year-old woman with a history of a liver transplant presented with altered mental status and seizures. MRI brain revealed bilateral parieto-occipital T2 hyperintensities. EEG showed bilaterally independent *(shown in underlines)* periodic sharp waves/spike waves (BIPDs) that are more pronounced on the right.

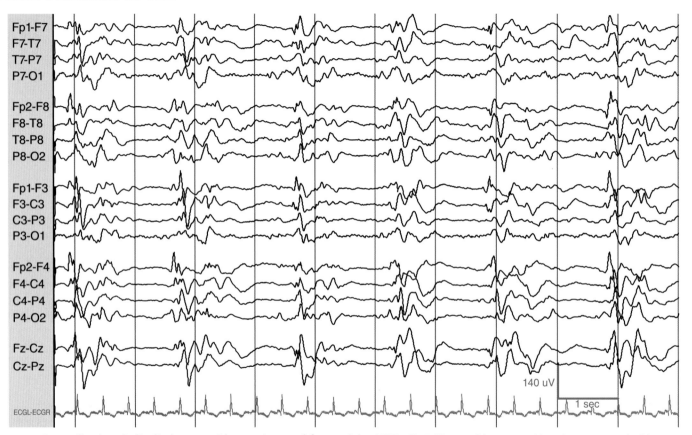

FIGURE 4.17 Generalized periodic discharges with superimposed fast activity (GPD+F). A 20-year-old woman with asthma presented with a severe asthma attack resulting in hypoxic-ischemic cerebral injury. EEG reveals generalized periodic spike/polyspike and wave discharges, with superimposed fast frequencies (GPD+F) occurring every 1.5–2 seconds. In between the discharges, the background is diffusely attenuated.

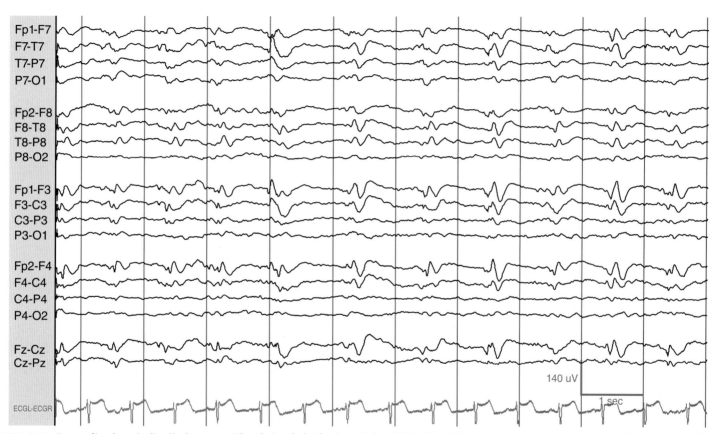

FIGURE 4.18 Generalized periodic discharges with admixed rhythmic activity (GPD+R). A 61-year-old man who was admitted with a subarachnoid hemorrhage. EEG revealed 1 Hz generalized periodic sharp waves with frequent admixed rhythmic delta activity (GPD+R) and an interval between complexes.

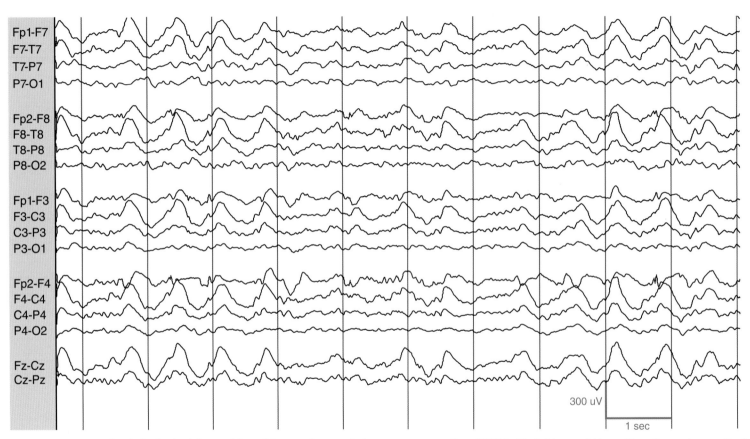

FIGURE 4.19 Generalized rhythmic delta activity with superimposed sharp waves or spikes (GRDA+S). A 14-year-old boy with autism and generalized epilepsy presented with altered mental status after a witnessed seizure. EEG revealed frequent generalized rhythmic delta waves with superimposed spike waves (GRDA+S).

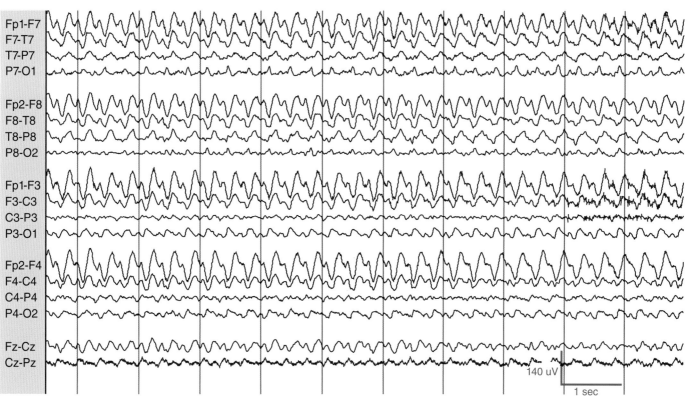

FIGURE 4.20 Generalized spike and slow wave (GSW). A 29-year-old man with generalized epilepsy and a psychiatric disorder presented with altered mental status and decreased verbal output after an electroconvulsive therapy (ECT) treatment. EEG revealed continuous sharp and slow waves occurring at 2.5 Hz. An antiseizure medication improved both the EEG and the patient's mental status. Though the frequency did not meet nonconvulsive status epilepticus (NCSE) on the basis of electrographic criterion alone (not more than 3 Hz), combined with altered mental status and improvement after medication, this pattern represents NCSE.

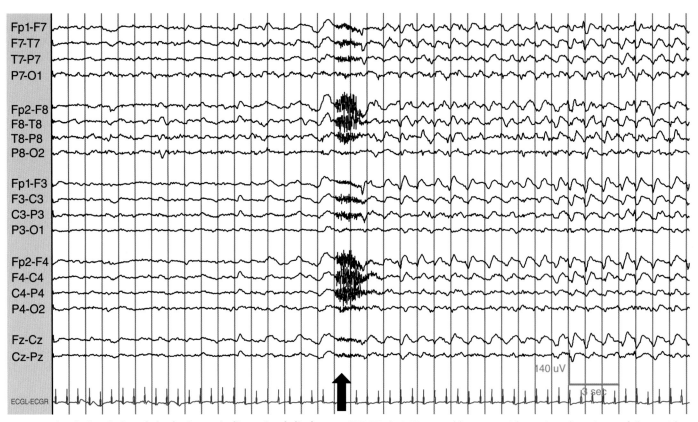

FIGURE 4.21 Stimulation-induced rhythmic, periodic, or ictal discharges (SIRPIDs). A 73-year-old woman with sepsis and respiratory failure. With a sternal rub *(arrow)*, there is development of generalized rhythmic delta activity with admixed sharp waves (GRDA+S) at 1 Hz. This pattern was repeatedly seen with stimulation, and each lasted about a minute.

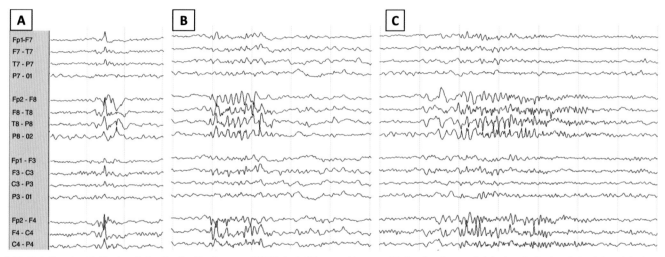

FIGURE 4.22 Brief potentially ictal rhythmic discharges (BIRDs). A 25-year-old man with focal epilepsy of right hemispheric origin. (A) A right hemispheric frontotemporal maximal sharp wave, (B) nonevolving BIRDs, and (C) evolving BIRDs.

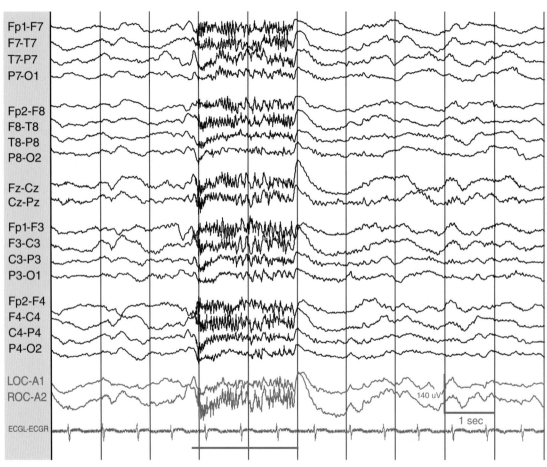

FIGURE 4.23 Generalized paroxysmal fast activity (GPFA), a subtype of brief potentially ictal rhythmic discharges (BIRDs). GPFA *(line)* in a 21-year-old woman with drug-resistant generalized epilepsy. There was no clinical correlate during this particular discharge.

Table 4.1 ACNS standardized critical care EEG terminology

ACNS Standardized Critical Care EEG Terminology 2021: Reference Chart

A. EEG Background

Symmetry	Background EEG frequency	PDR	Continuity	Reactivity	State Changes	Cyclic Alternating Pattern of Encephalopathy (CAPE)	Voltage	AP Gradient	Breach effect
Symmetric	Beta	Present Specify frequency	Continuous: <1% periods of suppression (<10 µV) or attenuation (>10µV but <50% of background voltage)	Reactive	Present with normal stage N2 sleep transients	Present	High ≥150 µV	Present	Present
Mild asymmetry <50% Voltage OR 0.5–1 Hz Frequency	Alpha	Absent		Unreactive	Present but with abnormal stage N2 sleep transients	Absent	Normal ≥20 to <150 µV	Absent	Absent
Marked asymmetry ≥50% Voltage OR >1 Hz Frequency	Theta	Unclear	Nearly continuous: 1–9% periods of suppression attenuation	SIRPIDs only	Present but without stage N2 sleep transients	Unknown/unclear	Low 10 to <20 µV	Reverse	Unclear
	Delta		Discontinuous: 10–49% periods of suppression or attenuation	Unclear	Absent		Suppressed <10 µV		
Localization of Bursts (G/L/Bl/Ul/Mf)	If Burst-suppression or Burst-attenuation then specify if:		Burst-suppression or Burst-attenuation: 50–99% periods of suppression or attenuation	Unknown					
Highly Epileptiform Bursts (Present or Absent)									
Identical Bursts (Present or Absent)			Suppression: >99% periods of suppression or attenuation						

(Continued)

Table 4.1 ACNS standardized critical care EEG terminology—cont'd

B. Sporadic Epileptiform Discharges	C. Rhythmic and Periodic Patterns (RPPs)	
Prevalence	**Main term 1**	**Main term 2**
Abundant ≥1/10s	**G** *Generalized* - Optional: Specify frontally, occipitally, or midline predominant; or generalized, not otherwise specified.	**PD** *Periodic Discharges*
Frequent ≥1/min but <1/10s	**L** *Lateralized* - Optional: Specify unilateral, bilateral asymmetric, or bilateral asynchronous - Optional: Specify lobe(s) most involved or hemispheric	**RDA** *Rhythmic Delta Activity*
Occasional ≥1/h but <1/min	**BI** *Bilateral Independent* -Optional: Specify symmetric or asymmetric - Optional: Specify lobe(s) most involved or hemispheric	**SW** *Spike and Wave* *OR* *Polyspike and Wave OR* *Sharp and Wave*
Rare <1/h	**UI** *Unilateral Independent* - Optional: Specify unilateral, bilateral asymmetric, or bilateral asynchronous for each pattern - Optional: Specify lobe(s) most involved	
	Mf *Multifocal* - Optional: Specify symmetric or asymmetric -Optional: Specify lobe(s) most involved or hemispheric	

Table 4.1 ACNS standardized critical care EEG terminology—cont'd

Major modifiers										Minor modifiers			
Prevalence	Duration	Frequency	Phases[1]	Sharpness[2]	Voltage (Absolute)	Voltage (Relative)[3]	Stimulus Induced or Stimulus Terminated	Evolution[4]		Onset	Triphasic[5]	Lag	Polarity[2]
Continuous ≥90%	Very long ≥1h	4 Hz	>3	Spiky < 70 ms	High ≥150 µV	>2	SI *Stimulus Induced*	Evolving		Sudden ≤3 s	Yes	A-P *Anterior-Posterior*	Negative
		3.5 Hz	3			≥2	ST *Stimulus Terminated*	Fluctuating		Gradual >3 s	No		Positive
Abundant 50–89%	Long 10–59 min	3 Hz		Sharp 70–200 ms	Medium 50–149 µV							P-A *Posterior-Anterior*	
		2.5 Hz	2				Spontaneous only	Static					Dipole
Frequent 10–49%	Intermediate duration 1–9.9 min	2 Hz	1	Sharply contoured >200 ms	Low 20–49 µV		Unknown					No	Unclear
		1.5 Hz											
Occasional 1–9%		1 Hz			Very low <20 µV								
	Brief 10–59 s	0.5 Hz		Blunt >200 ms									
Rare <1%		<0.5 Hz											
	Very brief <10 s												

Plus (+) Modifiers
No +
+F   *Superimposed fast activity – applies to PD or RDA only*   **EDB** *(Extreme Delta Brush): A specific subtype of +F*
+R   *Superimposed rhythmic activity – applies to PD only*
+S   *Superimposed sharp waves or spikes, or sharply contoured – applies to RDA only*
+FR   *If both subtypes apply – applies to PD only*
+FS   *If both subtypes apply – applies to RDA only*

NOTE 1: Phases: Applies to PD and SW only, including the slow wave of the SW complex
NOTE 2: Sharpness and Polarity: Applies to the predominant phase of PD and the spike or sharp component of SW only
NOTE 3: Relative voltage: Applies to PD only
NOTE 4: Evolution: Refers to frequency, location or morphology
NOTE 5: Triphasic: Applies to PD or SW only

Table 4.1 ACNS standardized critical care EEG terminology—cont'd

Brief Potentially Ictal Rhythmic Discharges (BIRDs)	Ictal-Interictal Continuum (IIC)
Focal (including L, Bl, Ul or Mf) or generalized rhythmic activity >4 Hz (at least 6 waves at a regular rate) lasting 20.5 s to <10 s, not consistent with a known normal pattern or benign variant, not part of burst-suppression or burst-attenuation, without definite clinical correlate, and that has at least one of A, B or C below:	1. Any PD or SW pattern that averages >1.0 Hz but ≤2.5 Hz over 10 s (>10 but ≤25 discharges in 10 s); OR 2. Any PD or SW pattern that averages ≥0.5 Hz and ≤1 Hz over 10 s (≥5 and ≤10 discharges in 10 s), and has a plus modifier or fluctuation; OR 3. Any lateralized RDA averaging >1 Hz for at least 10 s (at least 10 waves in 10 s) with a plus modifier or fluctuation; AND 4. Does not qualify as an ESz or ESE.
Definite BIRDs feature either: A. Evolution ("evolving BIRDs") OR B. Similar morphology and location as interictal epileptiform discharges or seizures in the same patient	
Possible BIRDS are C. Sharply contoured but without (a) or (b) above	

Reprinted with permission from Hirsch, L.J., Fong, M.W.K., Leitinger, M., et al., 2021. American Clinical Neurophy siology Society's standardized critical care EEG terminology: 2021 version. J. Clin. Neurophysiol. 38(1), 1–29.

Further reading

Garcia-Morales, I., Garcia, M.T., Galan-Davila, L., et al., 2002. Periodic lateralized epileptiform discharges: etiology, clinical aspects, seizures, and evolution in 130 patients. J. Clin. Neurophysiol 19(2), 172–177.

Gaspard, N., Manganas, L., Rampal, N., et al., 2013. Similarity of lateralized rhythmic delta activity to periodic lateralized epileptiform discharges in critically ill patients. JAMA Neurol 70(10), 1288–1295.

Hirsch, L.J., Claassen, J., Mayer, S.A., et al., 2004. Stimulus-induced rhythmic, periodic, or ictal discharges (SIRPIDs): a common EEG phenomenon in the critically ill. Epilepsia 45(2), 109–123.

Hirsch, L.J., Fong, M.W.K., Leitinger, M., et al., 2021. American Clinical Neurophysiology Society's standardized critical care EEG terminology: 2021 version. J. Clin. Neurophysiol 38(1), 1–29.

Kane, N., Acharya, J., Benickzy, S., et al., 2017. A revised glossary of terms most commonly used by clinical electroencephalographers and updated proposal for the report format of the EEG findings. Clin. Neurophysiol. Pract. 2, 170–185.

Leitinger, M., Trinka, E., Gardella, E., et al., 2016. Diagnostic accuracy of the Salzburg EEG criteria for non-convulsive status epilepticus: a retrospective study. Lancet Neurol 15(10), 1054–1062.

Rodriguez Ruiz, A., Vlachy, J., Lee, J.W., et al., 2017. Association of periodic and rhythmic electroencephalographic patterns with seizures in critically ill patients. JAMA Neurol 74 (2), 181–188.

Yoo, J.Y., Rampal, N., Petroff, O.A., et al., 2014. Brief potentially ictal rhythmic discharges in critically ill adults. JAMA Neurol 71(4), 454–462.

Yoo, J.Y., Jetté, N., Kwon, C.S., et al., 2021. Brief potentially ictal rhythmic discharges and paroxysmal fast activity as scalp electroencephalographic biomarkers of seizure activity and seizure onset zone. Epilepsia. 62(3), 742–751.

When evaluating a new patient, the first line of inquiry for the clinician is, "Is this a seizure?" There are many seizure mimics, including parasomnias, syncope, transient ischemic attacks, and psychogenic nonepileptic seizures (PNES). A seizure is defined by the International League Against Epilepsy (ILAE) as "a transient occurrence of signs and/or symptoms due to abnormal excessive or synchronous neuronal activity in the brain." If the event in question is a seizure, the next line of inquiry is, "Is the onset of the seizure generalized, focal, or unknown?" According to the ILAE, generalized epileptic seizures begin at "some point within and rapidly engaging, bilaterally distributed networks. Such bilateral networks can include cortical and subcortical structures, but not necessarily include the entire cortex. Generalized seizures can be asymmetric." Focal epileptic seizures begin "within networks limited to one hemisphere. They may be discretely localized or more widely distributed." In some cases, there can be more than one seizure focus, which makes the epilepsy multifocal. Focal seizures can spread to involve both hemispheres; hence the epilepsy type pertains to the onset and not the propagation pattern. The electrographic representation of a seizure is often similar between individuals (e.g., temporal lobe seizures from hippocampal sclerosis or absence seizures). Electrographic seizures always disrupt the background; they generally evolve from faster frequencies to slower frequencies, and the shape of the waves (morphology) often changes over the course of the seizure, most commonly becoming higher in amplitude. Multiple seizures from the same focus in the same individual will often have very similar patterns. Table 5.1 delineates different seizure types and the EEG patterns associated with each seizure type.

The next question is whether or not an individual has epilepsy. Epilepsy is a disease of the brain defined by any of the following conditions: (1) at least two unprovoked (or reflex) seizures occurring >24 hours apart; (2) one unprovoked (or reflex) seizure and a probability of further seizures similar to the general recurrence risk after two unprovoked seizures (at least 60%); or (3) the diagnosis of an epilepsy syndrome. This means that even if an individual has a history of six seizures, but they all occurred in the setting of hypoglycemia, this individual does not have epilepsy. Conversely, if a child has a single seizure and the EEG shows centrotemporal spikes, then by both criteria #2 and #3, this child has epilepsy (self-limited epilepsy with centrotemporal spikes [SeLECTS]).

Following are brief discussions of nine important epilepsy syndromes along with the principal electrographic findings. An epilepsy syndrome refers to identifiable disorders based upon multiple defining characteristics including but not limited to age of onset, EEG characteristics, and seizure type(s). These syndromes have implications for treatment and prognosis. Table 5.2 provides a list of most of the epilepsy syndromes as defined by the ILAE, along with salient clinical and electrographic features.

Infantile epileptic spasms syndrome (IESS)

This serious illness typically has its onset between 3 and 12 months, and nearly always before the age of 2 years. The triad consists of infantile spasms, hypsarrhythmia on EEG, and developmental regression. The typical spasm consists of a sudden, brief flexion movement of the body, with flexion of the neck and abduction of the arms. Extension of the neck

Table 5.1 Seizure types and associated EEG patterns

	Clinical characteristics	EEG findings during the seizure
Generalized seizures		
Generalized tonic-clonic (GTC)	During the tonic phase, there is loss of consciousness and full body stiffening, often accompanied by a loud cry. In the clonic phase, there is active rhythmic jerking.	Generalized fast activity (>10 Hz) that increases in amplitude and decreases in frequency during the tonic phase, with spikes and slow waves during the clonic phase (Fig. 5.1).
Typical absence	Impairment of awareness for several seconds without loss of body tone. Sudden onset and cessation. Can have eyelid fluttering and eyes may drift upward. No postictal phase. Duration from 5 to 20 seconds.	Regular and symmetric generalized, usually 3 Hz, spike and slow wave complexes (Fig. 4.7).
Atypical absence	Impairment of awareness, often with insidious onsets and offsets. Can have an atonic component. Duration from 5 to 30 seconds.	Diffuse, sometimes irregular, spike and wave <2.5 Hz. Can be asymmetric.
Myoclonic absence	Rhythmic 2.5–4 Hz jerks, usually of the shoulders, arms, and legs during the absence seizure. Can have perioral jerks and an underlying tonic component. Duration is up to 60 seconds.	Regular and symmetric generalized 3 Hz spike and slow wave complexes.
Eyelid myoclonia	The first component is spasmodic 4–6 Hz blinking (eyelid myoclonia), often followed by mild impairment in consciousness. Seizures triggered with eye closure in the presence of light or with photic stimulation. Can have a subtle tonic component. Brief; each seizure lasts for seconds.	Generalized 3–6 Hz spike and polyspike and wave discharges that are triggered by eye closure or flickering light.
Myoclonic	Brief (<100 ms), involuntary, shocklike, often irregular, jerking of the body. Can affect the whole body or just a part. Consciousness is typically not impaired.	Epileptic myoclonus is usually time locked to a generalized polyspike, which is followed by a wave (Figs. 5.2 and 5.3). Myoclonus may not have an EEG correlate.
Myoclonic-atonic	Brief myoclonic jerk followed by atonia (loss of muscle tone). Duration of myoclonic-atonic seizure is 1–2 seconds.	Myoclonic jerk correlates with a generalized polyspike; atonia correlates with the after going slow wave (Fig. 5.4).
Myoclonic-tonic	A myoclonic jerk or cluster of myoclonic jerks followed by a tonic seizure. Rare.	Myoclonic jerk correlates with a generalized spike, and tonic component may correlate with low-voltage fast activity.
Myoclonic-tonic-clonic	Begins with a cluster of myoclonic jerks often with preserved consciousness before becoming a tonic-clonic seizure.	Myoclonic jerks correlate with generalized spikes or polyspikes followed by generalized fast activity characteristic of the tonic phase and bursts of spikes and slow waves in the clonic phase.

Table 5.1 Seizure types and associated EEG patterns—cont'd

	Clinical characteristics	EEG findings during the seizure
Tonic	Sudden onset of a rigid increase in muscle tone, often with stereotyped posturing of the limbs lasting from seconds to minutes. More frequent from sleep. Can be subtle (eye elevation) or massive. Autonomic features are common.	Low-voltage fast activity, which may increase in amplitude and decrease in frequency (Fig. 5.5).
Clonic	Generalized clonic seizures are rare, consisting of loss of consciousness and bilateral 1–3 Hz rhythmic jerks, with the jerk lasting for <100 ms. A clonic seizure differs from myoclonus in that it is rhythmic (each jerk being *a clone* of the prior jerk). Frequency diminishes but amplitude of jerk does not. Lasts from minutes to hours.	Fast activity >10 Hz or occasional spike and wave pattern.
Atonic	A sudden loss or decrease of muscle tone, which may be confined to a body part (head), or diffuse, leading to falls.	Electrodecrement, polyspike and wave, or low-amplitude fast activity.
Focal seizures		
Focal seizures	Seizure manifestation depends on the area of the brain that is affected. People may be aware or have impaired awareness. Onset can be motor (limb clonus, hyperkinetic, automatisms) or nonmotor (autonomic, behavioral arrest, cognitive, emotional or sensory). Focal seizures can spread and become a tonic-clonic seizure.	EEG can show rhythmic activity of varying morphologies from the brain region that is seizing (Figs. 5.6 and 5.7). In seizures that do not recruit at least 6 cm^2 of cortex, the EEG may show no change from the background on a scalp recording.
Unknown		
Epileptic spasm	Onset of this seizure type is typically before the age of 1 year. Spasms are brief contractions of the axial muscles and can be clinically described as extensor, flexor, or mixed. In a mixed spasm, there may be extension of the legs, abduction of the arms, and flexion of the neck. Spasms cluster around sleep transitions. Movement is usually symmetric. Consistent asymmetry implies a possible focal lesion.	The background EEG shows a high-voltage chaotic pattern known as hypsarrythmia. The EEG during a spasm can demonstrate a diffuse slow wave followed by electrodecrement, electrodecrement alone, or generalized paroxysmal low-amplitude fast activity (GPFA) (Fig. 5.8).

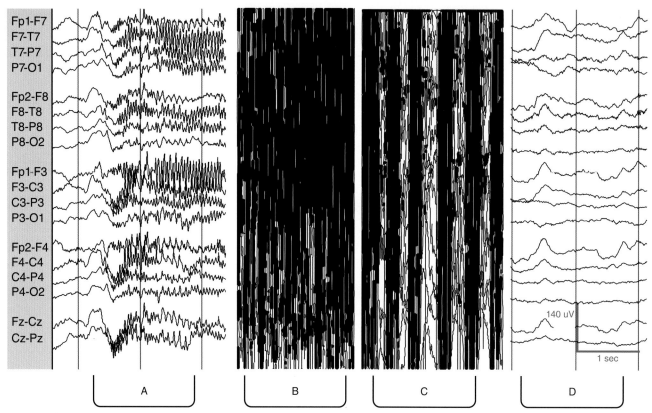

FIGURE 5.1 Generalized tonic-clonic (GTC) seizure. A 27-year-old woman with generalized tonic-clonic seizures. (A) There is diffuse rhythmic fast activity at the seizure onset. (B) The patient becomes tonic, and the EEG is entirely obscured by muscle artifact. (C) Clonic activity follows with characteristic rhythmic muscle artifact. (D) After the seizure, there is postictal slowing. The entire seizure lasted 64 seconds.

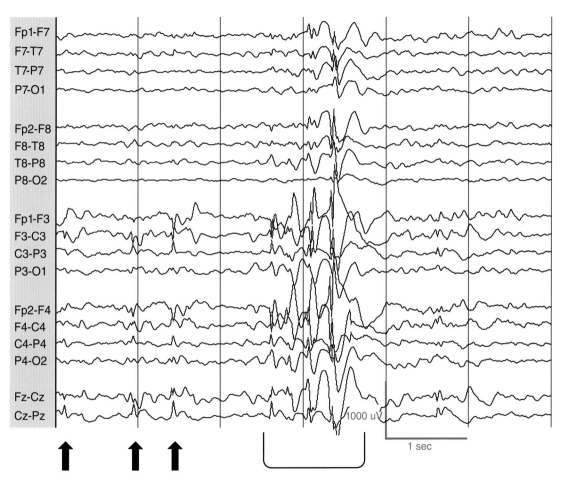

FIGURE 5.2 Myoclonic epilepsy of infancy (MEI). A 4-year-old boy with myoclonus since 8 months of age. A bilateral synchronous burst of high-amplitude 4 Hz polyspike and wave *(bracket)* is more prominent in the parasagittal region for 0.5 seconds and then becomes diffuse. A subtle myoclonic shoulder jerk was captured 100 ms after the last spike. *Arrows* show sporadic spikes, maximal in the parasagittal chain.

1000 uV

1 sec

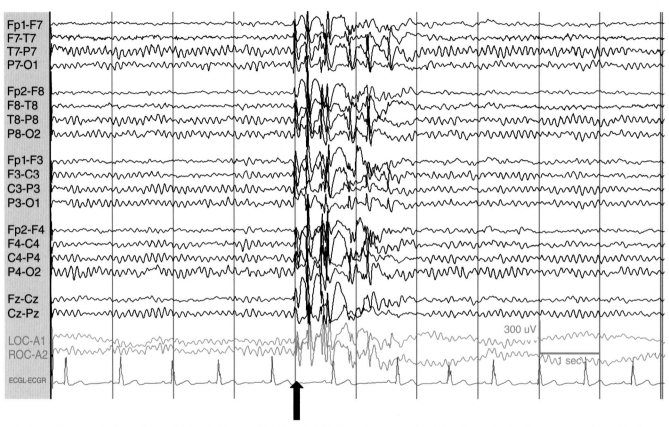

FIGURE 5.3 Juvenile myoclonic epilepsy (JME). A 17-year-old girl with JME. Generalized irregular 4 Hz spike and polyspike and wave *(arrow)* in the setting of a normal background. A jerk was reported by the technician during this discharge.

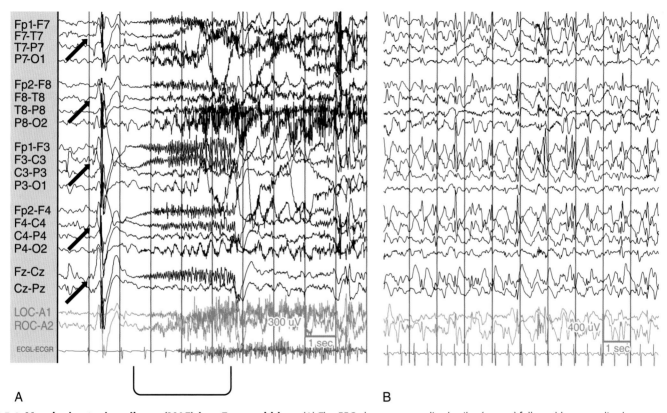

A

B

FIGURE 5.4 Myoclonic-atonic epilepsy (MAE) in a 7-year-old boy. (A) The EEG shows a generalized spike *(arrows)* followed by generalized paroxysmal fast activity (GPFA) *(bracket),* and then rhythmic slowing and admixed muscle artifact. (B) After this seizure, he became stuporous, drooling, and ataxic. EEG was consistent with a spike-wave stupor (absence status epilepticus) with continuous high-amplitude 1–2 Hz spike and wave complexes. Mental status improved with ASM management.

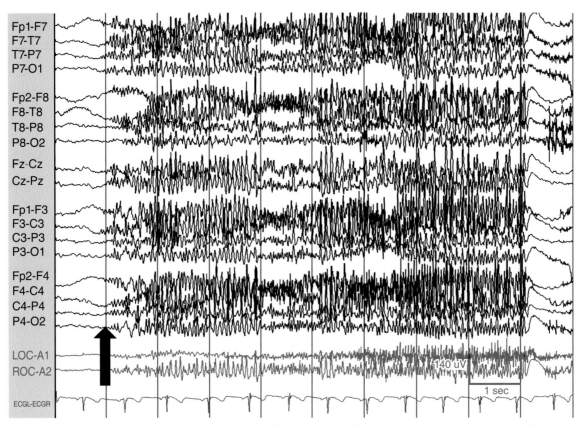

FIGURE 5.5 **Tonic seizure.** A 56-year-old male with developmental delay and tonic seizures. Diffuse beta activity *(arrow)* and admixed EMG artifacts are present for 8 seconds. Clinically correlates with eye opening and subtle raising of his arms.

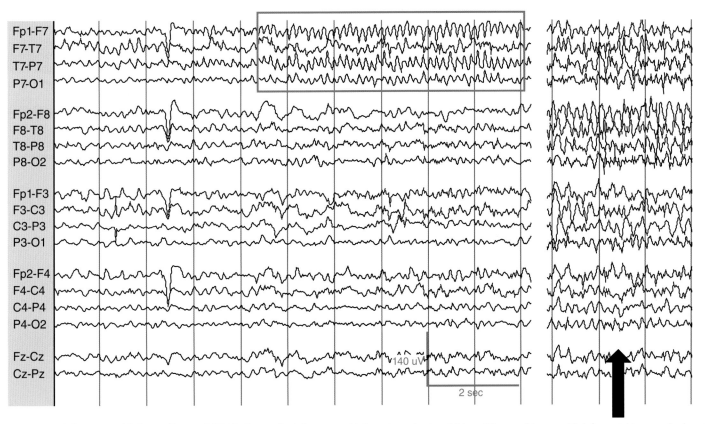

FIGURE 5.6 Mesial temporal lobe epilepsy (MTLE). Onset of a left temporal lobe seizure (rectangle) in a 58-year-old man with left mesial temporal sclerosis (MTS) and schizophrenia. *Rectangle* shows rhythmic left temporal theta activity. After 30 seconds, there is diffuse rhythmic activity of mixed frequencies *(arrow)*.

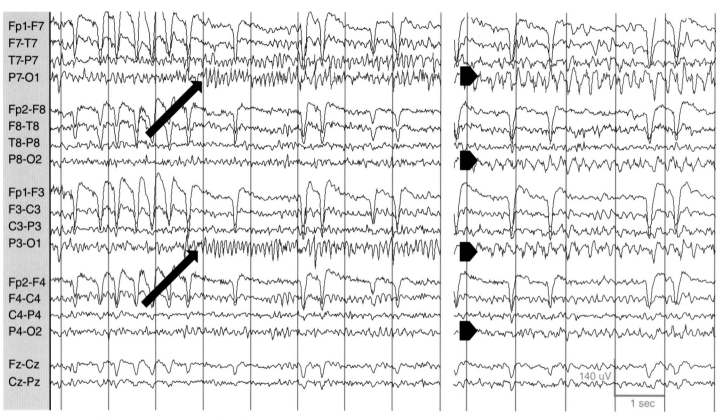

FIGURE 5.7 Occipital lobe seizure. A 21-year-old girl with Sturge–Weber syndrome, a left-sided port wine stain, and left posterior leptomeningeal angiomatosis. Onset of her left occipital seizure *(arrow)* with rhythmic alpha (mimicking a well-organized PDR!) evolves into bilateral occipital theta activity *(arrowhead)* with admixed spikes. Patient reports seeing a rainbow at onset.

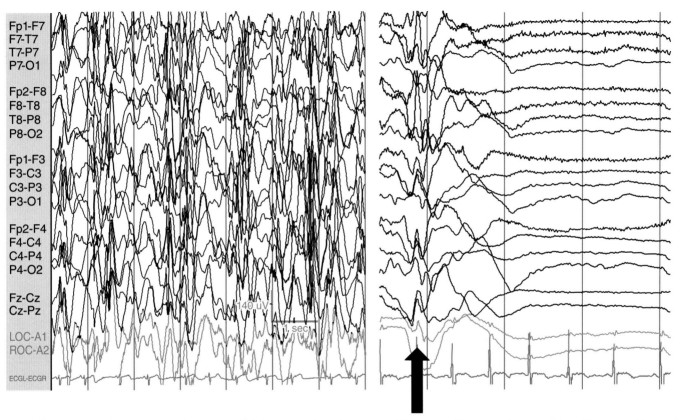

FIGURE 5.8 Infantile epileptic spasm syndrome (IESS). A 4-month-old previously normal baby boy with the development of infantile spasms. Hypsarrythmic background with high-amplitude, poorly organized, chaotic-appearing brain waves. A synchronous slow wave correlates with his clinical spasm *(arrow)* and is followed by electrodecrement.

Table 5.2 Epilepsy syndromes and other epilepsies

Syndrome Age of Onset	Clinical	EEG
Neonates and infancy		
Self-limited epilepsy of neonates and infants		
SeL(F)NE Days 2–7 of life	Usually unilateral clonic seizures but can be apneic. Neurologically normal. Autosomal dominant, de novo mutation thought to be responsible for lack of family history in some. 10%–15% progress to epilepsy. Multiple gene loci, usually a potassium channel.	Normal background. Theta pointu alternant pattern (theta runs with admixed sharp waves) and multifocal spikes can be seen.
SeLFNIE Day 2–7 months	Brief focal clonic or focal tonic seizures. Developmental milestones are normal. Often autosomal dominant. Often, sodium or potassium channel mutations are seen.	Normal background. Can be focal discharges and background slowing.
SeLIE 3–20 months	Seizures with behavioral arrest, automatisms; these often cluster and can secondarily generalize. Most common mutation is in PRRT2; sodium and potassium channel mutations also seen. Remits about 1 year after onset.	Normal background; may have midline spikes during slow sleep.
Febrile seizures + (FS+) (part of GEFS+) <6 months or lasts >6 years	Febrile seizures are the most common seizure type. May have afebrile seizures of multiple types. Neurologically normal. Usually autosomal dominant, responsive to ASM, and resolves by puberty.	Normal background. May have generalized spike and wave interictally.
MEI 4 months–3 years	Myoclonic seizures, occasionally myoclonic-atonic seizures. 30% have febrile seizures. Most neurologically normal. Aggressive treatment is postulated to help with overall development. Typically remits by age 6.	Normal background. Myoclonus is associated with generalized spike and polyspike discharges (Fig. 5.2).
Developmental and Epileptic Encephalopathies (DEE) of Neonates and Infants		
EIDEE (previously separated into Ohtahara and early myoclonic encephalopathy) Birth to 3 months	Tonic seizures, myoclonus, and severe encephalopathy. Focal, intractable seizures. Drug resistant. Poor prognosis. Often with genetic mutations, metabolic abnormalities, and/or structural abnormalities.	Burst suppression pattern. Multifocal spikes. Tonic seizures correlate with high-frequency, low-voltage fast activity. Myoclonus may have a spike-wave correlate.

Table 5.2 Epilepsy syndromes and other epilepsies—cont'd

Syndrome Age of Onset	Clinical	EEG
EIMFS <12 months, typically 3 months	Unprovoked bilateral independent multifocal prolonged focal seizures that are intractable and followed by neurological deterioration. Infants are normal at onset. Usually a KCNT1 mutation.	Normal background at onset and then deteriorates. Multifocal spikes between seizures. Seizures with multifocal electrographic onsets.
IESS (previously West syndrome) 1–24 months, typically 3–12 months	Infantile spasms, developmental regression. Commonly progresses to LGS. Often treated with ACTH, corticosteroids, or vigabatrin.	Hypsarrhythmia (chaotic, high amplitude, with multifocal epileptiform discharges). Diffuse slow or sharp wave with electrodecrement, electrodecrement alone, or GPFA during a spasm (Fig. 5.8).
DS 1–20 months, typically 3–9 months	Heat-sensitive bilateral tonic-clonic seizures, hemiconvulsions, myoclonic seizures, atypical absence, ataxia, and neurological decline. Majority have SCN1A mutation.	Normal background at onset of disease, which worsens over time. Focal and generalized spikes interictally.
Childhood		
Self-Limited Epilepsy (SeLFE) of Childhood		
SeLECTS (previously benign epilepsy with centrotemporal spikes) 3–14 years, typically 7 years	Rare, usually nocturnal seizures with unilateral facial sensations and movements. Can generalize. Normal neurologically. Typically remits by age 16.	Normal background. Abundant bilateral or unilateral centrotemporal spikes activated by sleep (Fig. 4.12).
SeLEAS (previously known as Panayiotopoulos syndrome) 1–14 years, typically 3–6 years	Rare nocturnal seizures with autonomic features (vomiting, pallor, syncope) and eye deviation. Often prolonged. Neurologically normal. Remits in 1–2 years. Can evolve into SeLECTS. Rarely can evolve into EE-SWAS.	Normal background. EEG variable with occipital, centrotemporal, parietal, and even generalized spikes. Discharges activate with sleep, eye closure, or darkness.
COVE (previously known as Gastaut syndrome) 1–19 years, typically 8–9 years	Frequent brief seizures during wakefulness, with visual elementary hallucinations, often with postictal migraine. Neurologically normal. Minority (5%–10%) will develop recurrent epilepsy.	Normal background. Mostly occipital spikes and sharp waves, activated by sleep, with eye closure or darkness (Fig. 4.6).
POLE 1–50 years, typically 4–17 years	Strong female preponderance. Seizures induced by photic stimulation or video games. Seizures with visual phenomena; can be lights or formed visual hallucinations.	Normal background. Occipital spikes and spike and wave facilitated by eye closure, photic stimulation, sleep, and sleep deprivation.

(Continued)

Table 5.2 Epilepsy syndromes and other epilepsies—cont'd

Syndrome Age of Onset	Clinical	EEG
Generalized epilepsy presenting in childhood		
EMAtS 6 months–8 years, typically 2–6 years	Myoclonic-atonic seizures, myoclonus, absence, bilateral tonic-clonic, and tonic seizures. Neurologically normal at onset. Developmental prognosis improves if seizures are controlled. About two-thirds of children achieve remission usually before age 3.	Background can be normal at onset. Interictal EEG can show generalized epileptiform potentials and parietal theta. Can go into status epilepticus after a GTC seizure (Fig. 5.4).
CAE 2–13 years, typically 4–10 years	Absence seizures. Neurologically normal. Majority will remit.	Normal background. Can have occipitally predominant, generalized rhythmic delta activity. Interictal generalized spikes or spike fragments. Seizures show 3 Hz spike and wave (Fig. 4.7).
EEM (previously Jeavon syndrome) 2–14 years, typically 6–8	Eyelid myoclonia +/– absence seizure induced by eye closure and photic stimulation. Drug resistant. Blue lens may improve seizure control. Infrequent GTC seizures. Lifelong condition.	Normal background. Brief 3–6 Hz irregular generalized polyspike and wave. Induced by eye closure and photic stimulation.
EMA 1–12 years, typically 7 years	Daily absence seizures, with myoclonus superimposed on tonic arm abduction. GTC, atonic, and absence seizures can also be present. Usually neurologically normal. Cognitive function preserved with seizure control. Often drug resistant.	Normal background. Interictal EEG with generalized 3 Hz spike and polyspike and wave.
Development and Epileptic Encephalopathies (DEE) of Childhood		
LGS 1–8 years, typically 3–5 years	Multiple seizure types, including tonic (most common), myoclonic, GTC, absence, atonic, and focal. Cognitive impairment. Drug resistant.	Background with slow spike and wave (1.5–2.5 Hz) (Fig. 5.9). MISF and PFA can be seen.
DEE-SWAS or EE-SWAS (previously known as Landau-Kleffner or epileptic encephalopathy with continuous spike-wave in sleep) 2–12 years, typically 4–5 years	Seizures can be atypical absence, GTC, atonic, and partial seizures. Primary clinical concern is often neuropsychological and behavioral changes. Can have language and motor regression. Can have thalamic lesions. Can have a genetic basis (GRIN2A). Prognosis is variable.	EEG shows almost continuous 1.5–2 Hz spike and wave in non-REM sleep, often >50% of slow wave sleep (Fig. 5.10). Can be diffuse, focal, or multifocal. In wake, epileptiform features are not continuous.

Table 5.2 Epilepsy syndromes and other epilepsies—cont'd

Syndrome Age of Onset	Clinical	EEG
FIRES (a form of NORSE) Typical 2–17 years, typically 8 years	Febrile illness typically 2 weeks to 24 hours before superrefractory status epilepticus. Acute phase of status epilepticus usually followed by DRE. Prognosis variable but can be poor.	Abnormal EEG background with slowing, multifocal discharges, delta brush. Seizures are usually focal or multifocal.
HHE <4 years	Onset with a prolonged, often febrile hemiconvulsion, followed by flaccid hemiplegia, which does not entirely resolve. Subsequent drug resistant focal epilepsy with cognitive impairment. MRI shows edema, followed by atrophy of the involved hemisphere. Prognosis poor.	Focal slowing and epileptiform potentials on the involved side.
Adolescence–adult		
Generalized epilepsy presenting in adolescence		
JAE 8–20 years, typically 9–13 years	Absence seizures, most with GTC seizures as well. Neurologically normal. Treatment is often lifelong.	Same as CAE (above).
JME 10–24 years	Myoclonic seizures, often in the morning. Can have GTC and absence seizures. Neurologically normal. Typically drug responsive but usually requires lifelong medication.	Normal background. Interictally, majority will have 4–6 Hz generalized polyspike and spike discharges (Fig. 5.3).
GTCA 5–40 years, typically 10–25 years	GTC seizure within 1–2 hours of awakening. Neurologically normal. Usually requires lifelong treatment.	Normal background. Generalized 3–5.5 Hz spikes and polyspikes, predominantly in sleep.
Developmental and epileptic encephalopathy of adolescence		
PMEs Variable onset	Heterogeneous group of disorders with myoclonus as a seizure type and typically a progressive course. (See Table 5.3 for more detail.)	Background may be normal at onset but worsens over time. Interictal EEG can show generalized and focal spikes (Fig. 5.11). Large somatosensory or visual evoked potentials.

(Continued)

Table 5.2 Epilepsy syndromes and other epilepsies—cont'd

Syndrome Age of Onset	Clinical	EEG
Variable age		
Focal epilepsy of variable age onset		
SHE Variable, typically 11–14	Focal motor seizures with hypermotor or hyperkinetic or tonic semiology. Movements are often large amplitude, complex with thrashing, pedaling, or pelvic thrusting possible. Usually neurologically normal. 30%–45% with daytime seizures. Includes genetic (autosomal dominant SHE), structural, and acquired causes.	Normal background. May have anterior spikes. Seizures often are surface negative.
FFEVF Infancy to adult	Each individual has a single focus, but family members may have different foci. Neurologically normal. Responsive to treatment. Autosomal dominant.	Normal background. May have focal epileptiform potentials interictally.
Epilepsy with auditory features (ADEAF) Infancy to adult	Focal seizures with buzzing, ringing, or sudden inability to understand language. Neurologically normal. Responsive to treatment. Can be a mutation in the LGI1 gene.	Background normal. Minority have focal temporal epileptiform potentials interictally. Ictal EEG shows temporal onset.
Etiology-specific epilepsy syndromes		
MTLE-HS	Typical auras include rising epigastric sensation, déjà vu, or fear. Focal seizures with impaired awareness and automatisms. Neurologically normal individuals, but some cognitive decline can occur with prolonged epilepsy. Often refractory to medical treatment.	Background may show focal slowing from involved temporal lobe. The majority have interictal anterior temporal sharp waves or spikes. Ictal EEG will often show rhythmic theta or alpha from the involved temporal lobe (Fig. 5.5).
RS 1 to adult, typically 6 years old	EPC and other focal seizures. Progressive hemiplegia and cognitive decline. Drug resistant. Hemispherectomy or hemispherotomy can be considered for seizure control.	EEG shows focal slowing and epileptiform potentials on the affected side (Fig. 5.12). EPC is often surface negative.
Gelastic seizures with hypothalamic hamartoma Variable, typically <12 months	Gelastic seizures are brief and frequent, with bursts of laughing or giggling; can secondarily generalize. Neurologically normal at onset but at risk of deterioration.	Background normal at onset. Can worsen. Interictal spikes are rare and can be focal or generalized. Seizures are typically surface negative.

Table 5.2 Epilepsy syndromes and other epilepsies—cont'd

Syndrome Age of Onset	Clinical	EEG
Other conditions with epileptic seizures		
FS 6 months–6 years, typically 18–24 months	Seizures occurring in the setting of a high fever. Can be simple (<15 minutes, generalized) or complex (>15 minutes, focal, abnormal neurological examination, and/or recurrent seizure within 24 hours). Family history common. Slight increased risk of developing epilepsy.	Background normal.
Reflex epilepsies	Syndrome in which *all* seizures are precipitated by sensory stimuli. Syndromes can involve multiple forms of photosensitivity, as well as reading, music, and startle. Can occur in neurologically normal and abnormal individuals.	These epilepsies can either be focal or generalized, with either normal or abnormal backgrounds (Fig. 2.11).
Epilepsies that do not fit into any of the above diagnostic categories	These include epilepsies caused by malformations of cortical development, neurocutaneous syndromes, tumors, infections, trauma, angiomas, perinatal insults, strokes, and epilepsies of unknown cause.	EEG depends on a particular cause. Seizures can be focal or generalized. Background can be normal or abnormal.

ACTH, Adrenocorticotropic hormone; *ASM*, antiseizure medication; *CAE*, childhood absence epilepsy; *COVE*, childhood occipital visual epilepsy; *DEE*, developmental and epileptic encephalopathies; *DEE-SWAS/EE-SWAS*, developmental and/or epileptic encephalopathy with spike-wave activation in sleep; *DRE*, drug-resistant epilepsy; *DS*, Dravet syndrome; *EEM*, epilepsy with eyelid myoclonia; *EIDEE*, early infantile DEE; *EIMFS*, epilepsy of infancy with migrating focal seizures; *EMA*, epilepsy with myoclonic absences; *EMAtS*, epilepsy with myoclonic-atonic seizures; *EPC*, epilepsia partialis continua; *FFEVF*, familial focal epilepsy with variable foci; *FIRES*, febrile infection-related epilepsy syndrome; *FS*, febrile seizures; *GEFS+*, genetic epilepsy with febrile seizures plus spectrum; *GPFA*, generalized paroxysmal fast activity; *GTC*, generalized tonic-clonic; *GTCA*, generalized tonic-clonic seizures alone; *HHE*, hemiconvulsion-hemiplegia-epilepsy; *IESS*, infantile epileptic spasms syndrome; *JAE*, juvenile absence epilepsy; *JME*, juvenile myoclonic epilepsy; *KCNT1*, potassium sodium-activated channel subfamily T member 1; *LGI-1*, leucine-rich glioma-inactivated 1; *LGS*, Lennox–Gastaut syndrome; *MEI*, myoclonic epilepsy in infancy; *MISF*, multiple independent spike foci; *MTLE-HS*, mesial temporal epilepsy with hippocampal sclerosis; *NORSE*, new-onset refractory status epilepticus; *PFA*, paroxysmal fast activity; *PMEs*, progressive myoclonic epilepsies; *POLE*, photosensitive occipital lobe epilepsy; *SCN1A*, alpha subunit of the neuronal type 1 sodium channel; *SeLEAS*, self-limited epilepsy with autonomic seizures; *RS*, Rasmussen syndrome; *SeLECTS*, self-limited epilepsy with centrotemporal spikes; *SeLFE*, self-limited epilepsy; *SeLFNIE*, self-limited familial neonatal-infantile epilepsy; *SeLIE*, self-limited (familial) infantile epilepsy; *SeLNE*, self-limited (familial) neonatal seizures; *SHE*, sleep-related hypermotor (hyperkinetic) epilepsy.

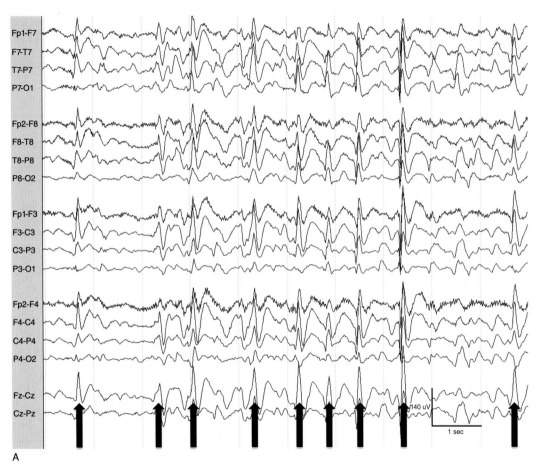

FIGURE 5.9 Lennox–Gastaut syndrome (LGS). (A) EEG shows frequent epochs with the characteristic slow 1.5–2 Hz spike and wave *(arrows)* pattern in this 44-year-old with LGS. There was no clinical correlate with these discharges.

A

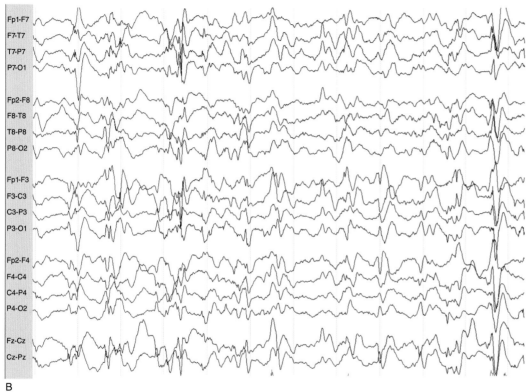

FIGURE 5.9, cont'd (B) Multiple independent spike foci (MISF) is another characteristic feature of LGS.

B

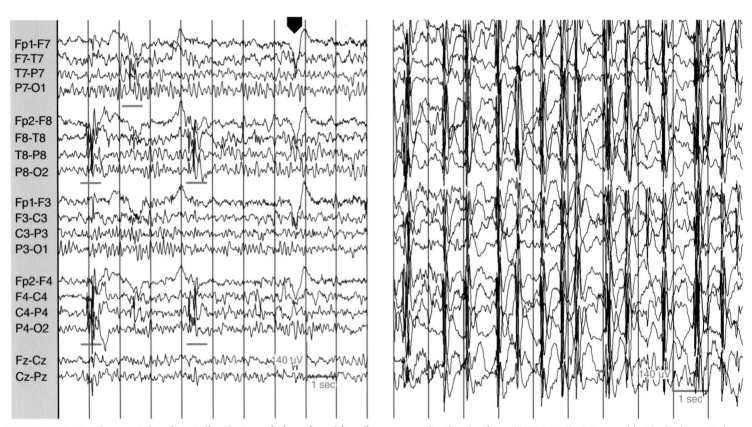

FIGURE 5.10 **Developmental and/or Epileptic Encephalopathy with spike-wave activation in sleep (DEE-SWAS).** A 6-year-old girl who began to have behavioral problems in school, developmental regression, and rare seizures. (A) Occasional bilateral independent spikes and polyspikes *(lines)* during wakefulness. Eye blink *(arrowhead)* and a PDR of 8 Hz are seen. (B) Continuous spike and wave during sleep (CSWS) with 1–2 Hz generalized spikes and polyspikes in sleep.

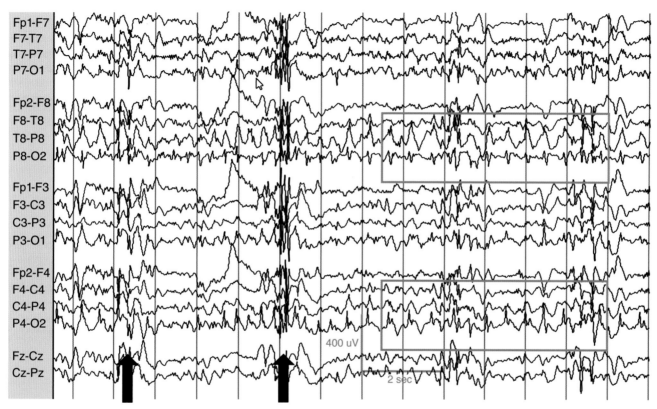

FIGURE 5.11 Progressive myoclonic epilepsy (PME), Lafora disease. A 16-year-old boy originally diagnosed with juvenile myoclonic epilepsy (JME) because of the presence of generalized polyspikes *(arrows)* but upon closer inspection, a number of features are inconsistent with JME, including a suboptimally organized and slow background with right posterior 2 Hz spike and wave *(rectangles)*.

and lower extremities may occur. The attacks are frequent, occurring in clusters around sleep transitions, and are associated with regression of milestones. Causes are multiple and include cerebral malformations (e.g., agyria, pachygyria), perinatal brain damage, tuberous sclerosis, and a variety of metabolic disorders (e.g., nonketotic hyperglycinemia). In about 15% of cases, no underlying cause can be identified.

The typical EEG feature is hypsarrhythmia, a more or less continuous, high-voltage (>350 µV), chaotic, slow wave pattern with frequent multifocal spikes and sharp waves (Fig. 5.8) Variations of this background pattern, termed modified hypsarrhythmia, are common. These include a burst suppression pattern, focal features (i.e., hemihypsarrhythmia), or slow waves without spikes. During the spasm, the most common correlate is a diffuse high-amplitude slow or sharp wave followed by electrodecrement (Fig. 5.8), but electrodecrement alone or low-amplitude fast activity can be seen. About half of the patients develop Lennox–Gastaut syndrome (LGS), and at least 80% develop cognitive impairment. Spasms are notoriously difficult to treat. Adrenocorticotropic hormone (ACTH) is highly effective and requires close monitoring due to the potential side effects of hypertension, cushinoid obesity, electrolyte disturbances, cardiomyopathy, or immunosuppression. Vigabatrin is another effective medication for spasms, particularly in children with tuberous sclerosis.

Dravet syndrome (DS)

Infants present with febrile seizures before the age of 2 years, typically around 6 months. Hot baths, infection, fever, and strong emotion all can trigger seizures. After several months, afebrile convulsions occur, followed by the development of myoclonic (onset 1–5 years) and atypical absence seizures. Hemiconvulsions with unilateral clonic activity are characteristic at the onset of the disease but less common in children older than the age of 3 years. Obtunded states with spike and wave and rare tonic seizures can be present. The infants may be normal at onset

but suffer from developmental delay and ataxia as the disease progresses. The EEG background is usually normal at onset and deteriorates over time. Interictally, there can be generalized and focal epileptiform potentials. The disease is associated in most cases with a mutation in the alpha subunit of the neuronal type 1 sodium channel (SCN1A). Due to the abundance of this channel on the inhibitory interneurons, any antiseizure medications (ASMs) that act on the sodium channel (including phenytoin, carbamazepine, and lamotrigine) can make the seizures worse and even propel the individual into status epilepticus. ASMs should be chosen that are broad spectrum AND not sodium channel blockers. The severity of the seizures correlates with the severity of neurological decline, and about 90% of children with Dravet are drug resistant. Newer treatments include cannabidiol, stiripentol, and fenfluramine for the treatment of Dravet as well as LGS.

Self-limited epilepsy with centrotemporal spikes (SeLECTS, previously benign rolandic or benign epilepsy with centrotemporal spikes)

This common epilepsy syndrome has its typical onset between the ages of 4 and 10. The disorder nearly always remits by age 16. Imaging studies are normal. The neurological examination is normal, as is the EEG background (well organized, with no focal or generalized slowing). There may be a family history of epilepsy or febrile seizures.

Common features during seizures include vocalization with guttural sounds, hypersalivation, unilateral oral/facial sensations, and clenching of the teeth. There may be hemifacial movements, hemiconvulsions, and even focal to bilateral tonic-clonic convulsions. Seizures typically occur upon falling asleep or upon awakening. Seizures are usually rare, but a small minority may have frequent events. Subtle neuropsychological difficulties have been encountered in children, typically involving attention and reading. These difficulties are thought to resolve when the interictal EEG improves in midadolescence.

Epileptiform discharges consist of sharp waves and/or spikes, often biphasic in configuration, occurring in the centrotemporal regions (C3/T3 and/or C4/T4) (Fig. 4.10). A horizontal dipole is often seen with negativity in the centrotemporal region and positivity in the frontal region. The discharges may occur in wakefulness but are usually markedly activated by drowsiness and sleep. Isolated sharp waves while awake often transform into grouped or periodic discharges during sleep and often alternate between the two hemispheres. There may be a left or right preponderance. Strictly unilateral discharges may also be seen. Rarely, some patients will have generalized discharges as well. Note that the EEG may contain many discharges, although few seizures have ever occurred. Interestingly, these discharges are seen in nearly 1% of children without a seizure disorder and it is estimated that only about 10% of children with centrotemporal sharp waves and spikes go on to develop epilepsy.

There is no universal agreement on treatment. Considering the self-remitting nature of the condition, the debate is whether to treat or not. ASMs are considered if seizures are more frequent or severe.

Lennox–Gastaut syndrome (LGS)

LGS has its onset in early childhood, usually around 3–5 years. The classic triad of LGS is cognitive impairment, multiple seizure types, and slow spike and wave (1.5–2.5 Hz) on the EEG. Seizure types include tonic (most common), atonic, myoclonic, focal seizures, and atypical absence. Status epilepticus is not rare and occurs in at least 50% of LGS patients. Typically, it is nonconvulsive, with atypical absence stupor and tonic seizures admixed.

About one-third of cases of LGS are of unknown cause, the remainder being due to congenital malformations, tuberous sclerosis, encephalitis, perinatal hypoxic brain damage, or other structural or metabolic disorders. Infants can first develop IESS in infancy and later evolve into LGS.

The EEG typically demonstrates a pattern of generalized slow spike-wave discharges at an average of 2 Hz (Fig. 5.9). In addition, multiple independent spike foci (MISF) and paroxysmal fast activity (PFA) are common.

Treatment of the seizures is difficult. ACTH, ketogenic diet, multiple ASMs, vagal nerve stimulators, responsive neurostimulation, deep brain stimulation, and corpus callosotomy have all been used, with variable success. As the clinician struggles to control the seizures, overmedication can occur, which can worsen mentation and balance.

Prognosis is generally poor, and the majority suffer from severe cognitive impairment, even if the seizures are eventually controlled.

Childhood absence epilepsy (CAE)

CAE usually makes its appearance at the time the child enters school, at about age 5 years, with a range between 4 and 8 years. These children are essentially normal, though with higher rates of attentional difficulties. The attacks themselves consist of staring episodes, with or without eye blinking, and generally are not longer than 10 seconds in duration. Minor automatisms appear in about 30% of cases, and occasional clonic or tonic features may be observed. Hyperventilation increases the likelihood of seizure occurrence, and pediatric neurologists routinely carry out the procedure in their offices in suspected cases. In the untreated state, hundreds of seizures may occur in a single day. There often is a family history of absence seizures, and twin studies have demonstrated a 75%–80% concordance for the seizures and the EEG trait.

The EEG is characteristic, demonstrating generalized 3 Hz spike and wave discharges (Fig. 4.7). During the seizure, the child is unresponsive but recovers immediately upon discharge cessation. At the same time, the normal background rhythms are restored, without evidence of postictal slowing. The background is typically normal in between discharges. However, bursts of occipitally predominant generalized rhythmic delta

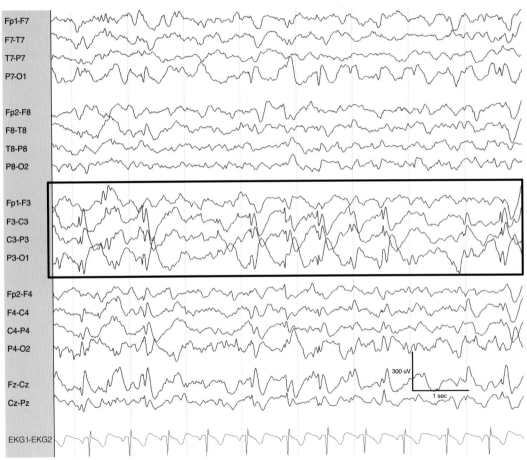

FIGURE 5.12 Rasmussen Syndrome (RS). A 7-year-old girl with Rasmussen syndrome. EEG shows abundant left parasagittal 1–2 Hz spike and wave *(rectangle)*, with some reflection on the right.

activity are not uncommon. During sleep, there is distortion of the generalized discharges—the frequency band declines, and polyspike-wave complexes are not uncommon.

A number of ASMs, including ethosuximide, valproate, lamotrigine, and topiramate, are likely to lead to complete seizure suppression. Agents such as carbamazepine and phenytoin, used for focal epilepsy, can worsen CAE. Numbers vary widely throughout the literature and 57%–74% of children with CAE will have a complete remission of their epilepsy in adolescence. If absence seizures are the only seizure type, about 80% of children will remit. If a child with absence seizures has a generalized tonic-clonic (GTC) seizure, the rate of remission is only 30%. Early institution of therapy improves the outcome. Of note, if a child with CAE is treated with ethosuximide and has a GTC seizure, another agent must be added. Ethosuximide is a great medication for absence seizures but does not control generalized seizures.

Juvenile myoclonic epilepsy (JME)
Patients with JME are typically adolescents who are neurologically normal with normal imaging. The first GTC seizure often occurs after a night of poor sleep and/or alcohol intake. There is frequently a history of myoclonic jerks in the morning, which may be bilateral or unilateral. Adolescents may feel that they are just clumsy in the morning and frequently drop spoons or fling their toothbrushes. A series of myoclonic jerks can lead to a GTC seizure. Absence seizures are seen in a substantial minority. There is a genetic predisposition. The interictal EEG demonstrates 4–6 Hz generalized spike and polyspike-wave discharges (Fig. 5.3). Thirty to 50% of patients with JME are photosensitive and their EEGs will show generalized spikes or polyspikes with photic stimulation. The seizures are usually well controlled with a broad-spectrum ASM. Limiting alcohol consumption and achieving regular sleep are cornerstones of therapy.

A particular feature of the syndrome should be emphasized: treatment is continued indefinitely, as relapse after discontinuation of ASMs occurs in the majority of patients.

Progressive myoclonus epilepsies (PMEs)
PMEs are a rare and heterogeneous group of disorders that are classified together because of their progressive and refractory nature and because myoclonus is one of the main seizure types. There is no cure for any of these disorders. Onset is typically in late childhood or early adolescence. In the beginning, the background EEG is typically normal, with sporadic generalized spike and polyspike discharges. The initial diagnosis may erroneously be JME. Over time, the background becomes slower and less organized. Individuals with PME have large somatosensory evoked potentials and visual evoked potentials, indicating the overall lack of inhibition to stimulation. Photosensitivity is common. Treatment is with any broad-spectrum ASM that is efficacious against myoclonus: valproic acid, benzodiazepines, levetiracetam, topiramate, and zonisamide, either alone or in combination, are all reasonable choices. Ketogenic diets have been tried as well. Clinical and electrographic features of the most common diseases in this category can be found in Table 5.3.

Mesial temporal lobe epilepsy with hippocampal sclerosis (MTLE with HS)
MTLE with HS accounts for about 20% of all adult epilepsy and typically causes focal seizures with an aura. The aura can be nausea, a rising epigastric sensation, intense fear, déjà vu, or an olfactory hallucination. This aura can pass after a few seconds to minutes, or it can develop into a focal impaired awareness seizure. At this stage, the eyes remain open, but the individual is not responding properly and there may be automatisms of chewing or picking movements. Autonomic features are common with sweating, pupillary dilatation, and heart rate changes. A focal to bilateral

Table 5.3 Progressive myoclonus epilepsies (PMEs)

PMEs	Disease characteristics
Unverricht–Lundborg disease (Baltic myoclonus) Before age 18, typically 7–13 years	Stimulus-sensitive myoclonus, GTC seizure, ataxia, and tremor. Cognition is relatively spared. Recessive mutation in EPM1 causing a cystatin B expansion. Most common PME.
Lafora disease Before age 20, typically 6–19 years	Stimulus-sensitive myoclonus, visual seizures, atonic seizures, GTC seizures, and blindness. EEG often has occipital spikes and occipital seizures, which is a distinguishing feature (Fig. 5.11). Progressive mental decline, with death often occurring within one decade after onset. Recessive mutations in either EPM2A (70%) or EPM2B (27%), causing a polyglucosan storage disorder.
MERRF Variable age of onset	Mitochondrial disorder characterized by myoclonus, generalized epilepsy, and ataxia. Can have myopathy, diabetes, deafness, cognitive decline, external ophthalmoplegia, and neuropathy. EEG shows giant somatosensory potentials and photosensitivity. MRI may show cortical atrophy and low signal in basal ganglia. May be sporadic or inherited; most (90%) caused by mutations in MT-TK. Muscle biopsy shows ragged red fibers in vast majority.
NCL Typically 4–7	Multiple disease subtypes. Children develop visual loss, GTC seizure, subtle myoclonus, psychiatric features, and later, dementia. Death within 10 years of diagnosis is common. Autosomal recessive disorder with different genes depending on subtype, all causing abnormal amounts of lipopigments in lysosomes. MRI is abnormal.
Sialidosis type 1 Variable age of onset	GTC seizure and an intention tremor begin in adolescence or adulthood. Cognitive decline, spasticity, ataxia, and a painful neuropathy can all occur. May have a cherry red spot on examination of fundus. Autosomal recessive disorder caused by deficiency of neuraminidase A, typically NEU1 mutation.
DRPLA Variable age of onset	Clinical features include epilepsy, parkinsonism, chorea, athetosis, myoclonus, and dementia. Frequently photosensitive. Rare autosomal dominant triplicate repeat disorder.

DRPLA, Dentato-rubro-pallido-luysian atrophy; *EPM*, epilepsy, progressive myoclonus; *GTC*, generalized tonic-clonic; *MERRF*, myoclonic epilepsy with ragged red fibers; *MT-TK*, mitochondrially encoded tRNA lysine; *NCL*, neuronal ceroid lipofuscinoses; *NEU1*, neuraminidase 1; *PMEs*, progressive myoclonus epilepsies.

tonic-clonic seizure (FTBTC) can occur. Seizures with impaired awareness are often followed by fatigue and confusion.

The interictal EEG in 90% of patients will show sporadic sharp waves and spikes from the affected side, often with phase reversal at the F7 (left) or F8 (right) electrodes. There may be some associated intermittent and often subtle temporal lobe slowing. The most common ictal pattern is rhythmic temporal theta or alpha activity within 30 seconds of symptom onset (Fig. 5.6). There may be some ipsilateral postictal slowing.

The etiology is not delineated in the majority of cases, but febrile seizures, particularly prolonged, and status epilepticus are possibly causative in some cases, as is antecedent traumatic brain injury.

Medication is the first-line treatment, but the clinician should be aware that 90% of patients with this condition will be drug resistant. Drug-resistant patients should be considered for surgical treatment. The majority of patients with refractory seizures due to HS will be free of disabling seizures after surgery and have a better quality of life.

Rasmussen syndrome (RS)

This is a rare epilepsy syndrome, which in the vast majority of cases presents in childhood. A typical case starts with the development of focal seizures (with or without secondary generalization) in an otherwise healthy child between the ages of 1 and 10. Status epilepticus is not an uncommon first manifestation. Epilepsia partialis continua (EPC), ongoing focal clonic motor seizures without impairment of consciousness, is a hallmark of the entity. As the disease develops, there is a progressive hemiparesis and cognitive decline. MRI early in the disorder may show focal hyperintense signal in the cortex of the affected side on T2 or FLAIR sequences. Later, there is progressive hemiatrophy. The EEG may show focal slowing in the abnormal hemisphere, as well as multifocal, usually but not always lateralized epileptiform potentials (Fig. 5.12). EPC often has no electrographic correlate. RS is difficult if not impossible to treat with ASMs. Surgical resection and/or disconnection (hemispherectomy/hemispherotomy) of the affected side can be an effective treatment for the seizures. Immunotherapy with intravenous immunoglobulin (IVIG), steroids, other immunosuppressants, and neuromodulation with responsive stimulation may be of benefit for seizure control and cognition in some cases, though further research is needed.

THE VALUE OF THE EEG IN EPILEPSY PROGNOSIS

Many clinicians place great value on the EEG when deciding whether or not to discontinue ASMs in seizure-free patients. Although it seems obvious that an epileptiform EEG should stay one's hand from discontinuing ASMs, the correlation between potential seizure recurrence and the presence of discharges is not consistent. Many studies have been published, with varying results. A benchmark for considering discontinuation is 2 years of seizure freedom, although this varies from 2 to 5 years, depending on the particular study.

In adults, a good rule of thumb is that after 2 years of seizure freedom, the patient has a 60% chance of remaining seizure-free after slow withdrawal of medication. The lack of epileptiform activity on the EEG means a better chance of success, but this is by no means a guarantee. Ongoing either generalized or focal spikes decrease the rate of success. If patients with generalized epilepsy continue to display generalized spike-wave discharges, the probability of seizure recurrence is relatively high. Note that even brief discharges of 1–2 seconds' duration are likely to correlate with very brief clinical lapses of which the patient is unaware. In this case, medication should be continued.

Multiple clinical circumstances increase the rate of relapse, including a diagnosis of JME or posttraumatic epilepsy, multiple seizures prior to control with ASMs, tonic-clonic seizures, polytherapy, and an abnormal neurological examination.

Other considerations are important, e.g., the patient's temperament and occupation (is driving required?). The issue must be discussed in detail with the patient, offering the pros and cons of discontinuation. Some patients do not want to take ASMs if not absolutely necessary and are willing to chance the possibility of seizure recurrence. Others are quite fearful of a possible seizure and are adamant about remaining on ASMs. As with all physician-patient interactions, a mutual understanding is essential for arriving at an individualized plan that is acceptable to both parties. The situation is different in children, as there is a good chance of "growing out of" some of the childhood-onset epilepsies.

Drug-resistant epilepsy (DRE)

Despite the development of numerous new ASMs, about 30% of patients are drug resistant. DRE means that the person continues to have seizures despite having tried at least two appropriate ASMs at therapeutic doses, either alone or in combination. It is important to refer patients in this category for surgical evaluation. Possible surgical interventions include laser ablation and resection of the seizure onset zone as well as neuromodulation with vagal nerve, deep brain, or responsive stimulation. Intracranial EEG is discussed in Chapter 6.

The EEG in seizure mimics

When seizures are possibly but not definitely the etiology of an event, the EEG is an indispensable tool in making an accurate diagnosis. Common seizure mimics in sleep are night terrors and somnambulism, both of which occur in slow-wave sleep. In adults, REM behavior disorder (RBD), with loss of the normal paralysis in REM sleep, leads to acting out of dreams. In RBD, the EEG shows REM sleep and events that can be hyperkinetic and are not particularly stereotyped. During breath-holding spells in children and in syncope in all ages, the EEG will show diffuse slowing but no underlying seizure activity (Fig. 5.13). Movement disorders, self-stimulatory behavior, confusional migraines, transient ischemic attacks, benign myoclonus of sleep, daydreaming, cataplexy, narcolepsy, and reflux (in infants) can all mimic seizures. For all of these, the EEG shows no underlying seizure.

The most frequently encountered mimic in the epilepsy monitoring unit is PNES. It is essential to capture the event in question with video EEG (VEEG) to make the diagnosis, as even in epilepsy, a normal EEG background is often seen between seizures. In addition, a significant minority of patients (percentages vary widely but approximately 10%–19%) will have both PNES and epilepsy. The same individual may have interictal spikes and events that are psychogenic. Any individual with events that are not controlled with ASMs should be brought in for EEG monitoring because the diagnosis has a profound impact on the approach to care: the events may be uncontrolled because the epilepsy is drug resistant, and a more aggressive approach is needed, or the events may be uncontrolled because the diagnosis is PNES and in this case, no ASMs are needed. Given the overlap between epilepsy and PNES, it is important to capture all known clinical events before discharging the patient off ASMs. The authors suggest both referral to psychiatry and continued neurological followup of patients with PNES. The neurological followup is to help reinforce the diagnosis of PNES and to prevent the reaccumulation of unnecessary and potentially harmful ASMs from other well-meaning but misinformed physicians.

PNES have some clinical characteristics that may be helpful: eye closure, asynchronous shaking, pelvic thrusting, erratic stopping and starting of movements with various amplitudes and frequencies, head shaking from side to side, and bilateral movements with preserved consciousness. While the EEG is often obscured during PNES by movement, if there are brief pauses, a normal PDR can be discerned. There is no postictal slowing after an event.

Beware; surface negative seizures in which the seizure activity is either too small (<6 cm^2 of activated cortex) or too distant from the recording electrodes can be mistaken for PNES. For example, EPC with ongoing focal motor activity is surface negative about 50% of the time. The movement is not suppressible and will often persist in sleep, which is key to

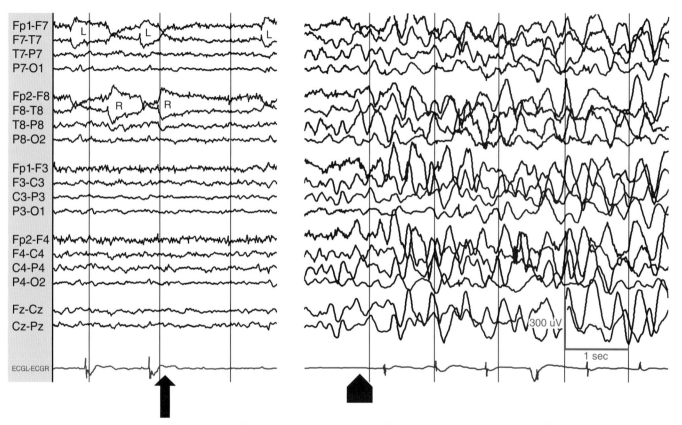

FIGURE 5.13 Pre-syncope due to asystole. A 14-year-old girl presents with episodes of feeling strange. EEG shows onset of asystole *(arrow)* which, after 15 seconds (not shown), is followed by diffuse theta and delta slowing *(arrowhead)* consistent with global hypoperfusion. Asystole resolves at the moment of diffuse cerebral slowing and there is no loss of consciousness. Additionally, lateral eye movement artifact is seen, with saccades to the right *(R)* and to the left *(L)*.

diagnosis. Frontal lobe seizures, which can be bizarre and hyperkinetic, are often surface negative, with no postictal slowing. These tend to be brief and highly stereotyped. When an event shows no EEG correlate, the video is not trivial, as the clinician must rely on a thorough knowledge of seizure semiology in order to make the right diagnosis.

Further reading

Gloss, D., Pargeon, K., Pack, A., et al., 2021. Antiseizure medication withdrawal in seizure-free patients: practice advisory update summary. Report of the AAN Guideline Subcommittee. Neurology 97 (23), 1072–1081.

Fisher, R.S., Acevedo, C., Arzimanoglou, A., et al., 2014. ILAE official report: a practical clinical definition of epilepsy. Epilepsia 55 (4), 475–482.

Hartman, A.L., Cross, J.H., 2014. Timing of surgery in Rasmussen syndrome: is patience a virtue? Epilepsy Curr 14, 8–11.

Hirsch, E., French, J., Scheffer, I.E., et al., 2022. ILAE definition of the idiopathic generalized epilepsy syndromes: position statement by the ILAE Task Force on Nosology and Definitions. Epilepsia 63 (6), 1475–1499.

Knight, E.M.P., 2020. Electroclinical syndromes of infancy. In: Wyllie, E. (Ed.), Wyllie's Treatment of Epilepsy: Principles and Practice, 7th ed. Lippincott Williams & Wilkins, Philadelphia, pp. 183–199.

Nickels, K., Shellhaas, R., Wyllie, E., et al., 2020. Electroclinical syndromes in childhood and adolescence. In: Wyllie, E. (Ed.), Wyllie's Treatment of Epilepsy: Principles and Practice, 7th ed. Lippincott Williams & Wilkins, Philadelphia, pp. 200–219.

Riney, K., Bogacz, A., Somerville, E., et al., 2022. International League Against Epilepsy classification and definition of epilepsy syndromes with onset at a variable age: position statement by the ILAE Task Force on Nosology and Definitions. Epilepsia. 63 (6), 1443–1474.

Specchio, N., Wirrell, E.C., Scheffer, I.E., et al., 2022. International League Against Epilepsy classification and definition of epilepsy syndromes with onset in childhood: position paper by the ILAE Task Force on Nosology and efinitions. Epilepsia. 63 (6), 1398–1442.

Steriades, C., Chauvel, P., Kotagel, P., 2020. Seizure types and semiology. In: Wyllie, E. (Ed.), Wyllie's Treatment of Epilepsy: Principles and Practice, 7th ed. Lippincott Williams & Wilkins, Philadelphia, pp. 145–160.

Tinuper, P., Bisulli, F., Cross, J.H., et al., 2016. Definition and diagnostic criteria of sleep-related hypermotor epilepsy. Neurology 86 (19), 1834–1842.

Varadkar, S., Bien, C.G., Kruse, C.A., et al., 2014. Rasmussen's encephalitis: clinical features, pathobiology, and treatment advances. Lancet Neurol 13 (2), 195–205.

DRUG-RESISTANT EPILEPSY

When people with epilepsy fail to have seizure freedom despite adequate trials of two tolerated, appropriately chosen, and appropriately used antiseizure medications (ASMs), their epilepsy is defined as drug-resistant epilepsy (DRE). About one-third of people living with epilepsy have DRE and, despite the development of many new ASMs, this rate has not significantly changed. People with DRE are at greater risk of suffering not only from their seizures and seizure-related injuries, but also from medication side effects, cognitive deterioration, decreased quality of life, and increased risk of sudden unexpected death in epilepsy (SUDEP). Surgical options have become less invasive and more varied in the last decade. Patients with DRE should be referred to a comprehensive epilepsy center for further evaluation and management. A list of comprehensive epilepsy centers in the United States can be found at https://www.naec-epilepsy.org/

PRESURGICAL WORKUP

The presurgical workup includes an admission for video-EEG (VEEG) to characterize the patient's seizures as well as an MRI protocolled for epilepsy to evaluate for structural abnormalities, however subtle. Neuropsychological testing can identify focal cognitive weakness that often colocalizes to the seizure onset zone (SOZ). For example a person with dominant temporal lobe epilepsy may have a deficit in verbal memory. In select cases, a PET scan, fMRI, Wada, magnetoencephalogram, or ictal single-photon emission computed tomography (SPECT) is used.

Most centers present cases at multidisciplinary conferences to integrate all of the history, physical examination, seizure semiology, EEG, imaging, and neuropsychological data to optimize an individualized plan for patients. This non-invasive work-up is often termed phase 1. Intracranial EEG monitoring is called phase 2.

INDICATIONS FOR INTRACRANIAL EEG

If an individual has a focal lesion that is concordant with VEEG and neuropsychological testing (for example, right mesial temporal sclerosis with right temporal seizures on VEEG and poor visual memory), then intracranial EEG is not needed. Either a right anterior temporal resection or a right mesial temporal laser ablation is a reasonable intervention. However, when noninvasive data lateralize but do not localize or localize but not lateralize (for example, in frontal lobe epilepsy), intracranial EEG is necessary to evaluate the epileptogenic zone. Other reasons that necessitate intracranial EEG are if the SOZ is in eloquent cortex or if noninvasive data are not concordant, suggesting a complex network. Finally, a previously failed epilepsy surgery may benefit from an intracranial EEG study.

Every intracranial EEG is tailored to the individual patient, with the goal of providing the information needed to make the next decision. A well-thought-out hypothesis of the patient's seizure network is crucial to designing intracranial electrode placement. With that in mind, the goal is to have electrode contacts in the SOZ as well as to define the borders of the SOZ. If the MRI is lesional and thought to be putative, the electrodes are often planned around the lesion.

INTRACRANIAL STUDY TYPES: STEREO-EEG VERSUS GRIDS AND STRIPS

Intracranial EEGs can be done as subdural grids, strips, and depth electrodes examination or as a stereo-EEG (SEEG) study. Grid placement requires a craniotomy and strip/depth electrodes may require additional burr holes (Fig. 6.1A). SEEGs are penetrating electrodes, placed with stereotactic techniques and preplanned trajectories, with lower morbidity (Fig. 6.1B).

Regardless of which kinds of intracranial EEGs are planned, one thing is common; you can only see what is going on in the electrodes you have. For example, a patient gets a feeling of suffocation (a typical insular aura) followed by déjà vu and the VEEG shows right frontotemporal onsets, an SEEG plan should include insular as well as mesial temporal contacts. If the SEEG fails to have contacts in the insula, the onsets may appear in the right hippocampus and amygdala, but any intervention in this area will not likely lead to seizure freedom. This point stresses the integration of the noninvasive data and careful planning. Table 6.1 suggests SEEG guidelines, depending on the type of epilepsy.

A grid is often used when the SOZ is suspected to be on the cortical convexity and particularly when there is a need to map language function. SEEG studies are uniquely suited to explore deeply located cortical areas such as the hippocampus, insula, cingulate, and deep-seated lesions like periventricular heterotopias and hypothalamic hamartomas. Additionally, SEEG is useful for bilateral exploration in cases with bilateral mesial temporal lobe epilepsy or nonlateralized frontal lobe epilepsy.

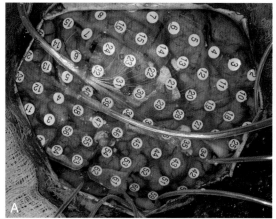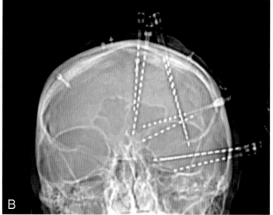

FIGURE 6.1 Intracranial studies. (A) Grid and (B) left-sided stereo-EEG (SEEG) implant.

Table 6.1 SEEG planning depending on type of epilepsy

Suspected localization	General sampling areas
Temporal lobe epilepsy	Mesial temporal structures (hippocampus and amygdala)
	Entorhinal cortex
	Middle temporal gyrus and basal cortex
	Superior temporal gyrus
	Temporal pole
	Insular cortex (floor)
Temporal lobe epilepsy involving extra-temporal or contralateral structures	Orbito frontal cortex
	Perisylvian region
	Temporoparietal junction
	Contralateral mesial temporal structures
Frontal lobe epilepsy (pre-liminary robust hypothesis in terms of lateralization and localization (anterior versus posterior, mesial versus dorso lateral) is mandatory)	Anterior frontal cortex
	Orbital cortex
	Cingulate gyrus
	Insula
	Posterior frontal cortex
	Supplementary motor area
	Motor cortex
	Consider temporal lobe coverage
Posterior epilepsy	Often require multilobar sampling, unilateral or bilateral, with particular concern for the pathways of propagation and the involvement of functional structures
Perisylvian epilepsy	Insula
	Opercula
Lesional epilepsy	Depends on the type of causal lesion
	One or several intralesional electrodes (except in vascular malformation or cystic lesion)
	Perilesional electrodes

SEEG, Stereo-EEG.

From Isnard J., Taussig D., Bartolomei F., et al., 2018. French guidelines on stereoelectroencephalography (SEEG). Neurophysiol. Clin. 48 (1), 5–13; Khoo, H.M., Hall, J.A., Dubeau, F., et al., 2020. Technical aspects of SEEG and its interpretation in the delineation of the epileptogenic zone. Neurol. Med. Chir. 60, 565–580.

INTRACRANIAL EEG

After intracranial EEG placement, postoperative imaging (MRI or CT scan coregistered to MRI) is done. Sampling frequency of intracranial EEG should be at least 256 Hz, though higher sampling rates >1000 will allow evaluation of high-frequency oscillations (HFOs). Typically, the high-frequency filter is left off as oscillations of higher frequency in an intracranial study are of interest and not artifact. The low-frequency filter works well at 0.5 Hz. Amplifier sensitivity needs to be lowered compared to scalp and often 50 μV/mm is used. The time base of 30 mm/s remains the same. To optimize the quality of the intracranial EEGs, the ground and reference electrodes should be intracranial as well. HFOs are important to visualize as they can help define the SOZ. In order to visualize HFOs, the low-frequency filter should be raised to 50 Hz and the high-frequency filter can be left off or raised as high as the software in the EEG program allows.

Both a referential and bipolar montage should be created. Similar to scalp EEG, two electrodes may have in-phase cancellation, and a referential montage is useful to appreciate the precise maxima.

The structure of the report is organized similar to that of the scalp EEG as described in Table 9.1. Clinical information should contain a description of the semiology of all of the patient's known seizure types. Next, the technical description needs to specify if this is an SEEG or grid/strip study, the number of electrodes, and their location. Be warned that there is no standard nomenclature in SEEG monitoring. Each SEEG lead contains between 5 and 18 contacts. Lower numbers (1, 2, 3) are most internal (i.e., hippocampus), whereas the higher numbers (10, 11, 12) are more external (i.e., lateral temporal lobe).

Each lead should be named and the location of the internal and external contacts should be identified on imaging and documented (Table 6.2). A thorough understanding of the 3D electrode array is necessary for

Table 6.2 Sample unilateral left (L) sided SEEG table

Electrode name and number of contacts	Internal contact	External contact
LmOlF 10	Mesial orbital	Lateral inferior frontal gyrus
LaCaS 10	Anterior subgenual cingulate	Anterior superior frontal gyrus
LmCpS 10	Mid-cingulate	Posterior superior frontal gyrus (note contacts 3-4 through leg motor)
LAgIT 10	Amygdala	Lateral anterior temporal, superior temporal gyrus
LHpIT 10	Hippocampus	Lateral midtemporal, middle temporal gyrus
LpTpT 10	Posterior mesial temporal, parahippocampal gyrus	Lateral posterior temporal, middle temporal gyrus
LaEiT 10	Anterior entorhinal	Anterior inferior temporal gyrus
LaImS 12	Anterior insula	Midsuperior frontal gyrus
LpIpM 12	Posterior insula	Supplementary motor area

SEEG, Stereo-EEG.

correct conceptualization and interpretation. At our institution, we name leads by location, with the first part of the abbreviation indicating the internal contacts and the last part of the abbreviation indicating the external contacts. For example, HplT is the name for the lead that goes from the **Hip**pocampus to the lateral Temporal lobe, with uppercase indicating the structure and lowercase typically indicating the position. Depending on the number of leads implanted, it can be challenging to display all contacts on one page for EEG reading. Constructing a montage that excludes contacts in white matter can make for more efficient reading.

Simultaneous scalp electrodes

At our institution, during all intracranial studies, we perform simultaneous scalp recordings. The simultaneous scalp electrodes corroborate that the intracranial seizures captured have the same pattern as previously captured VEEG seizures. In addition, for patients with push button events with no intracranial correlate, scalp EEG helps ensure that a seizure is not missed due to inadequate sampling (for example, in a unilateral intracranial study). Furthermore, we can determine how many of the patient's seizures are seen on scalp as many of the seizures are surface negative or have a delayed scalp onset.

Background

In intracranial EEG, many of the scalp landmarks are nowhere to be found. Posterior dominant rhythm and sleep architecture as we know it are absent. Typically, in wake, there are a mix of frequencies, and in sleep, the frequencies slow. White matter and unlayered gray matter like the amygdala tend to be flatter than parts of the brain with cortical layers like the hippocampus and neocortex (Fig. 6.2). Reader beware: physiologic activity intracranially is often sharply contoured and higher in amplitude and can be difficult to discern from epileptiform activity.

Focal slowing and/or attenuation can be seen in regions of dysfunction and should be commented on.

Interictal epileptiform abnormalities

Spikes, sharp waves, lateralized rhythmic delta activity (LRDA), lateralized periodic discharges (LPDs), and brief potentially ictal rhythmic discharges (BIRDs) will all be found in the intracranial EEG, often with a far greater frequency and spatial location than scalp (Fig. 6.3A). The frequency and morphology of the spiking can help characterize the SOZ. For example, continuous periodic discharges can indicate focal cortical dysplasia (Fig. 6.4C), whereas frequent low-amplitude spikes with admixed low-voltage fast activity (LVFA) can be seen in nodular heterotopia.

HFOs >80 Hz are a good indicator of the epileptogenic zone (Fig. 6.4D).

Seizures

The same principles for analyzing a scalp seizure apply to an intracranial seizure. The first step is to look at and describe the clinical semiology in detail. Then the EEG is examined, primarily for seizure onset location (Figs. 6.3C, 6.4C, and 6.5C). An onset with LVFA suggests the SOZ and, when localized to a few contacts, the prognosis for surgical cure is high. Low-frequency, high-amplitude spike and wave in the hippocampus is often seen with mesial temporal sclerosis (Fig. 6.3C). If the clinical onset precedes the EEG onset or if only slowing is seen, this suggests inadequate coverage of the SOZ.

BRAIN MAPPING DURING AN INTRACRANIAL STUDY

Electrical stimulation mapping (ESM) is one of the most fascinating procedures we get to do. ESM is done to answer particular questions, specifically to define eloquent cortex and to elicit a habitual seizure. ESM can define functional brain regions, particularly for motor and language,

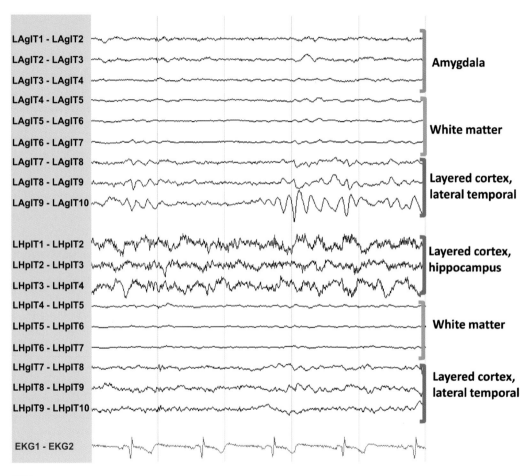

FIGURE 6.2 Stereo-EEG (SEEG). Two leads, one from the amygdala to the anterior lateral temporal lobe (AgIT) and the second from the head of the hippocampus to the midlateral temporal lobe (HpIT). Contacts in white and in the unlayered gray matter are lower in amplitude than contacts in layered gray matter.

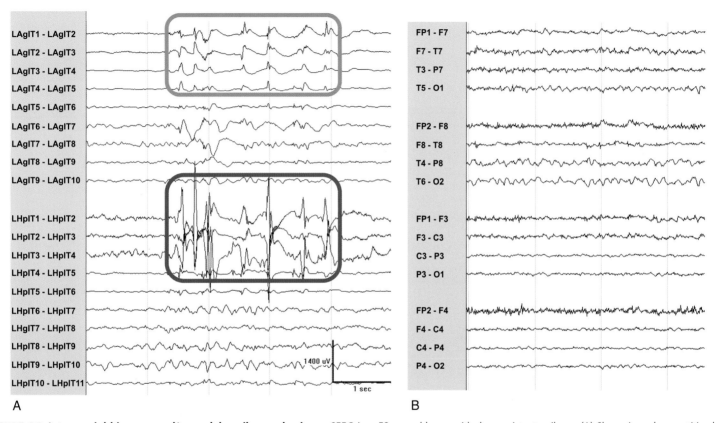

FIGURE 6.3 Intracranial hippocampal/amygdala spikes and seizure. SEEG in a 53-year-old man with drug-resistant epilepsy. (A) Shows irregular repetitive left hippocampal spikes and polyspikes *(blue rectangle)* also seen in the left amygdala but lower in amplitude *(orange rectangle).* (B) Simultaneous scalp EEG does not show any epileptiform potentials.

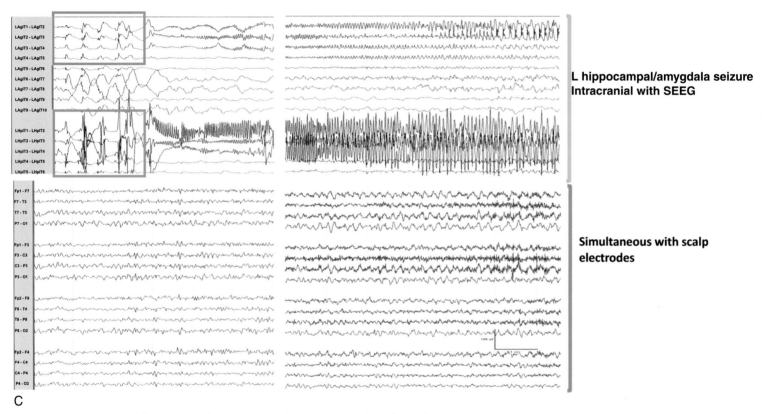

C

FIGURE 6.3, cont'd (C) A left hippocampal seizure starts with repetitive irregular spikes in the hippocampus *(blue rectangle)* and the amygdala *(orange rectangle),* followed by rhythmic beta activity. A seizure is seen on the scalp after a delay, with rhythmic theta maximal at the F7–T7 electrodes (flatter in this bipolar montage).

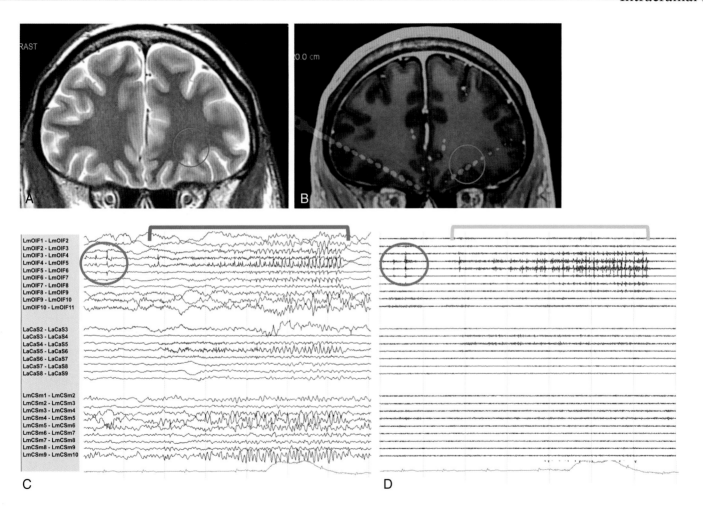

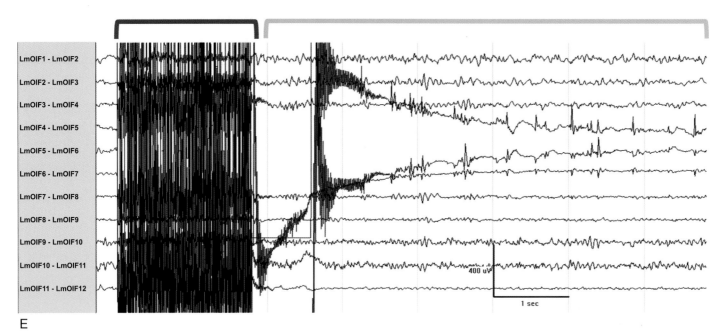

E

FIGURE 6.4 Intracranial EEG in sleep-related hypermotor epilepsy. A 38-year-old man with multiple seizures with nausea, a postnasal drip sensation, and a metallic taste, noted to have grimacing, pelvic thrusting, and leg movements. Bilateral study was done as VEEG was not clinically or electrographically lateralizable. (A) Coronal T2 MRI showing a subtle left orbitofrontal focal cortical dysplasia *(red circle)*. (B) SEEG with the bilateral mesial orbitofrontal to lateral frontal leads (bilateral mOlF). (C) Near-continuous low-amplitude periodic discharges were seen at LmOlF 3–6, characteristic of a focal cortical dysplasia. There is then an evolution *(red bracket)*, with a broader onset, maximal at LmOlF 3–6 *(red circle in B)* and LaCaS 4–6. The movement artifact in the EKG demonstrates that this was subtly clinical. (D) With the low-frequency filter set at 50 and the high-frequency filter off, the high-frequency oscillation (HFO) *(blue bracket)* can be seen and provides accurate localizing data. (E) During brain mapping, when high-frequency stimulation was delivered to the LmOlF 5 & 6 contacts *(purple bracket)*, the patient felt his typical focal aware seizure with a feeling of nausea and a postnasal drip sensation. The stimulation caused afterdischarges (repetitive spiking) at LmOlF4–7 *(orange bracket)*. He underwent focal resection of the lesion.

close to or in the epileptic focus that then must be avoided surgically to prevent dysfunction. ESM with subdural grids is considered the standard for language localization as the electrode contacts are contiguous and close enough that the boundaries can be mapped carefully for resective surgeries. Not all of the electrodes need to be stimulated.

There are varying protocols for ESM. A typical protocol is to stimulate an electrode pair (bipolar, juxtaposed electrodes) at 50 Hz for 1–5 seconds at various levels of current until an area is determined to be clear or involved. With high-frequency stimulation during SEEG, we typically do not exceed 4 mA. Lower-frequency stimulation may be used (5 or 10 Hz) and with this protocol, higher current intensities may be required. If there is a functional alteration, afterdischarges or a seizure, stimulation in that area

is stopped. For language testing, the patient performs a series of language tasks (counting, months of the year, auditory naming, visual naming, and repetition) during stimulation. Motor function is assessed by having the patient raise both arms supine and stick out their tongue. If near the leg area, the legs must be exposed. The patient is also asked to provide descriptions of any sensations they may experience. Causing seizures during ESM is common and typically the epileptologist will deliver brief (approximately 200 ms) bursts of stimulation to interrupt them. In addition, it is wise to have IV benzodiazepine nearby. The triggering of a *typical* aura or seizure helps to identify the epileptic network (Fig. 6.4E).

The report should document in detail the results at each electrode pair, including the maximal intensity reached; motor, sensory, or language

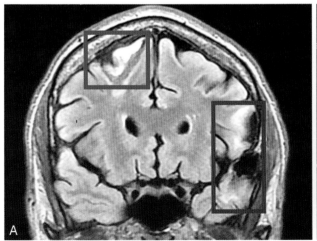
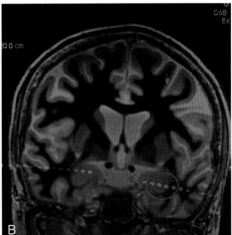

FIGURE 6.5 Intracranial EEG in posttraumatic epilepsy, with seizures causing asystole. A 30-year-old man with a remote left anterior temporal and inferior frontal brain injury secondary to head trauma (A, *brown rectangle*) developed seizures in which he would fall limply to the ground, recently sustaining a right frontal contusion (A, *blue rectangle*). Bilateral SEEG leads were placed. The *red circle* in B indicates the electrographic seizure onset in the left amygdala.

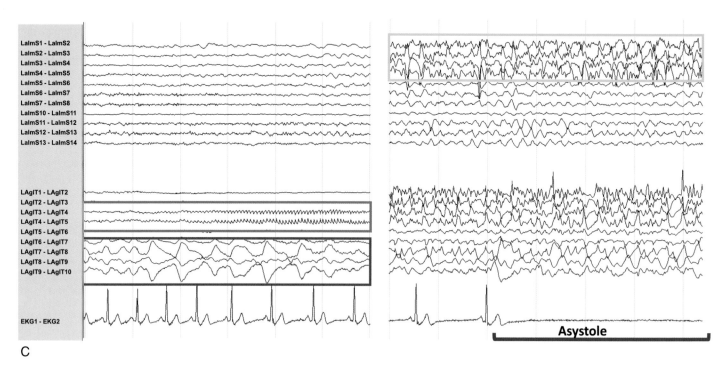

C

FIGURE 6.5, cont'd (C) The LalmS lead has the internal contacts in the left insula (1–5) and the external contacts in the middle frontal gyrus (12–14). The LAglT lead has the internal contacts (1–4) in the left amygdala and the external contacts in the anterior lateral temporal lobe (7–10). The anterior lateral temporal lobe showed continuous diffuse delta slowing as it was in the area of encephalomalacia *(green rectangle)*. The seizure onset is seen in the left amygdala *(red rectangle)*. When the seizure spread to the anterior insula *(yellow rectangle)*, the patient became asystolic, which lasted for 26 seconds and caused syncope. He was treated with a cardiac pacemaker as well as a left amygdala and anterior temporal resection, sparing the hippocampus. He has been seizure-free since.

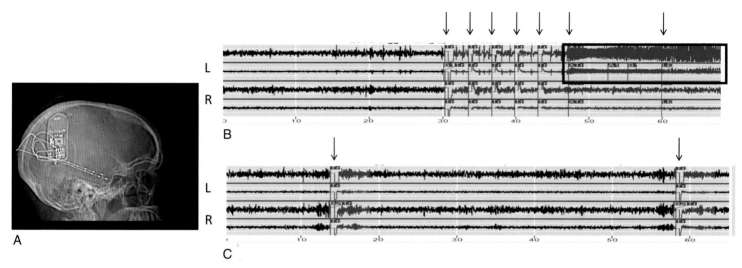

FIGURE 6.6 Responsive neurostimulation system (RNS). A 55-year-old woman with bilateral mesial temporal lobe epilepsy and bilateral hippocampal depth electrodes (A). Compressed EEG data from the left and right hippocampi. (B) The *blue* shows the detection onset of a possible seizure with multiple stimulations *(arrows)* delivered to stop the seizure. The stimulation fails and a clear left temporal seizure *(box)* is seen. (C) Two detections *(blue)* and stimulations *(arrows)* are depicted and a seizure does not develop.

findings; and whether the stimulation caused afterdischarges or a seizure. Finally, the conclusion should summarize the pertinent findings.

INTRAOPERATIVE ELECTROCORTICOGRAPHY (ECOG)

Intraoperative electrocorticography (ECoG) means monitoring direct brain activity in the operating room by a subdural grid or strip.

Intraoperative ECoG can be used to observe frequent interictal activity in order to adjust resection margins previously determined by the intracranial EEGs or determining the resection margins of a potentially epileptogenic MRI-visible lesion, such as a type II cortical dysplasia. Direct functional mapping can be done at the same time when resective surgery poses a risk for a motor-sensory, language, or visual deficit (within or in close proximity to the eloquent cortex). In these cases, the treatment team should ensure that the patient is able to be awake and communicative during the resective process.

RESPONSIVE NEUROSTIMULATION ELECTROCORTICOGRAPHY (ECOG)

With the responsive neurostimulation device (NeuroPace Inc.), in clinical use since 2013, we are now able to observe ECoGs of selected brain regions over long periods of time. The responsive neurostimulation system (RNS) device can connect two leads with four contacts on each one, which are placed in the patient's epileptogenic zone, for recording of ECoGs and delivering stimulation therapies (Fig. 6.6). This device is programmed to detect the individual's seizure onset pattern and deliver stimulation in an attempt to abort the seizure propagation. The device is indicated when the epileptogenic zone is not in a safe area for resection due to its function (eloquent cortex) or when there are two epileptogenic foci. The RNS system not only provides therapeutic effects but also has diagnostic value. For example, in cases of bilateral mesial temporal lobe epilepsy, with RNS electrodes placed in both medial temporal structures, the percentage of seizures from each side can be observed over an extended period. If the vast majority of seizures come from one side, an ablative procedure may be of great benefit. With this unprecedented opportunity to observe brain activity over long periods of time, we are now able to expand our understanding of epilepsy, such as seizure temporal dynamics (circadian and multidien patterns), as well as directly viewing an individual's response to certain medications.

Further reading

Baud, M.O., Kleen, J.K., Mirro, E.A., et al., 2018. Multi-day rhythms modulate seizure risk in epilepsy. Nat. Commun. 9 (1), 88.

Casale, M.J., Marcuse, L.V., Young, J.J., et al., 2022. The sensitivity of scalp EEG at detecting seizures – a simultaneous scalp and stereo EEG study. J. Clin. Neurophysiol. 39 (1), 78–84.

Frauscher, B., Ellenrieder, N., Zelmann, R., et al., 2018. Atlas of the normal intracranial electroencephalogram: neurophysiological awake activity in different cortical areas. Brain 141, 1130–1144.

Hirsch, L.J., Mirro, E.A., Salanova, V., et al., 2020. Mesial temporal resection following long-term ambulatory intracranial EEG monitoring with a direct brain-responsive neurostimulation system. *Epilepsia*. 61(3):408–420.

Isnard, J., Taussig, D., Bartolomei, F., et al., 2018. French guidelines on stereoelectroencephalography (SEEG). Neurophysiol. Clin. 48 (1), 5–13.

Khoo, H.M., Hall, J.A., Dubeau, F., et al., 2020. Technical aspects of SEEG and its interpretation in the delineation of the epileptogenic zone. Neurol. Med. Chir. 60, 565–580.

Quraishi, I.H., Mercier, M.R., Skarpaas. T.L., et al., 2020. Early detection rate changes from a brain-responsive neurostimulation system predict efficacy of newly added antiseizure drugs. *Epilepsia*. 61(1):138–148.

Young, J.J., Coulehan, K., Fields, M.C., et al., 2018. Language mapping using electrocorticography versus stereoelectroencephalography: a case series. Epilepsy Behav. 84, 148–151.

Zangaladze, A., Sharan, A., Evans, J., et al., 2008. The effectiveness of low-frequency stimulation for mapping cortical function. Epilepsia 49 (3), 481–487.

The EEG in other neurological and medical conditions and in status epilepticus

THE DEMENTIAS

There are many subtypes of dementias, and EEGs are nonspecific, often showing slowing of the posterior dominant rhythm (PDR), loss of the usual anterior beta activity, and a gradual increase in diffuse slowing. Nevertheless, certain EEG features can help with our understanding of the problem. For example, focal slowing is most prominent in the anterior regions in frontotemporal dementia. In its early stages, Alzheimer's disease may display little or no EEG abnormality. As the disease progresses, first, there is slowing of the PDR, which may eventually be lost entirely. Epileptiform discharges may appear later in the process and may be focal, generalized, or even periodic (Fig. 7.1). Note that clinical seizures, generalized or focal, become more common as dementia progresses—particularly in its late stages.

Multi-infarct dementia (MID) is difficult to differentiate from other types of dementias on clinical grounds as well as on EEG grounds. In MID, the record is more likely to display asymmetric features. This no doubt results from multiple small strokes in the course of the illness.

Creutzfeldt–Jakob disease (CJD) has distinctive EEG and clinical characteristics. The disease is rapidly progressive, with cognitive decline and parallel EEG changes. The background rhythms become fragmented and are destroyed. Diffuse slowing appears and increases. Later, the distinctive periodic sharp waves, often at 1 Hz, are recorded (Fig. 7.2). At first, the discharges may be more irregular and even focal, later becoming generalized and synchronous. Background activity decreases in amplitude. Eventually, the EEG is dominated by the periodic discharges, with no discernible background. Before death, there is a decline in and ultimate disappearance of the discharges, leaving an essentially featureless record. A clinical note: the appearance of periodicity is commonly associated with myoclonus. Although the periodic sharp waves are associated with myoclonus, they are not usually time locked with the myoclonus.

ISCHEMIC STROKE

Many patients presenting with acute ischemic stroke are relatively easy to diagnose on clinical grounds with respect to the history and physical examination. Note to our readers: the neurological examination still retains its importance! Others are less straightforward, and the clinician depends on an imaging study to aid in accurate diagnosis. In an acute cortical stroke, the CT of the brain may be normal, while the EEG shows a focal decrease of amplitude from a reduction of cortical electrical production (Fig. 7.3). Note that a similar voltage attenuation can be seen when there is an increase in fluid or blood between the cortex and the electrodes (e.g., subdural hematoma [SDH]). These two conditions are hard to differentiate just from an EEG. Asymmetry of beta rhythms with reduction of amplitude is the earliest and most sensitive indicator of cortical dysfunction or a local cortical lesion. Then polymorphic focal slow waves may appear in an area of reduced amplitude, suggesting that white matter under the cortex is involved as well. In some patients with acute infarction, epileptiform potentials (sharp waves and/or spikes) may be recorded. Furthermore, the EEG sometimes reveals a pattern of lateralized rhythmic delta activity (LRDA) or lateralized periodic discharges (LPDs).

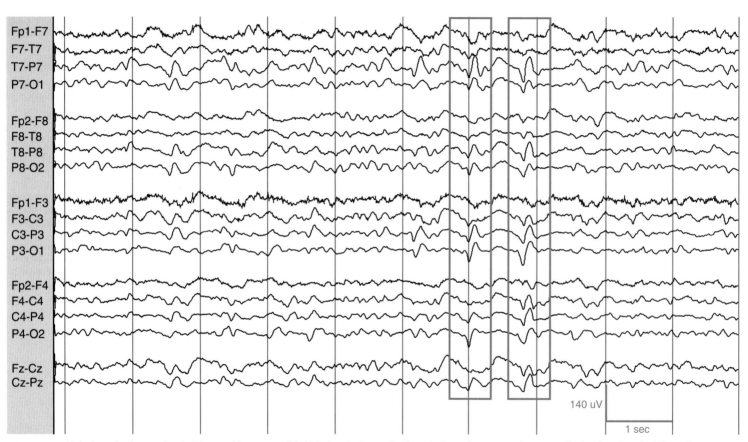

FIGURE 7.1 Alzheimer's dementia. A 90-year-old woman with Alzheimer's dementia. There is loss of posterior dominant rhythm (PDR) with diffuse slowing, most prominent over the posterior region. Generalized sharp waves are posteriorly predominant *(boxes)*.

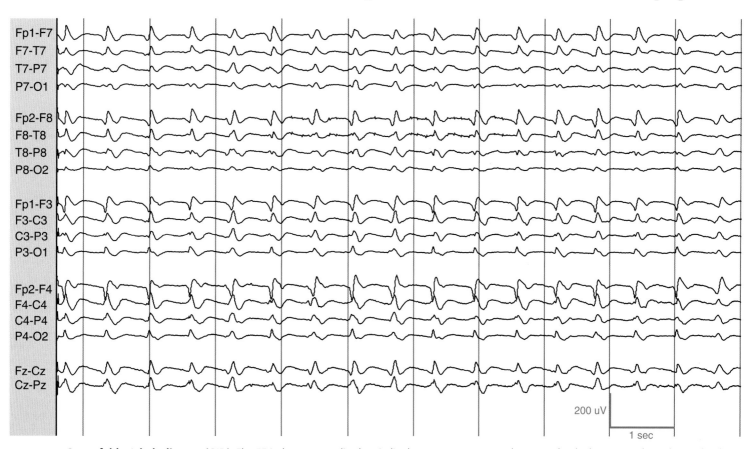

FIGURE 7.2 Creutzfeldt–Jakob disease (CJD). The EEG shows generalized periodic sharp waves at 1–2 Hz that are either biphasic or triphasic (generalized periodic discharge [GPD]) on a suppressed background in this 64-year-old woman with CJD.

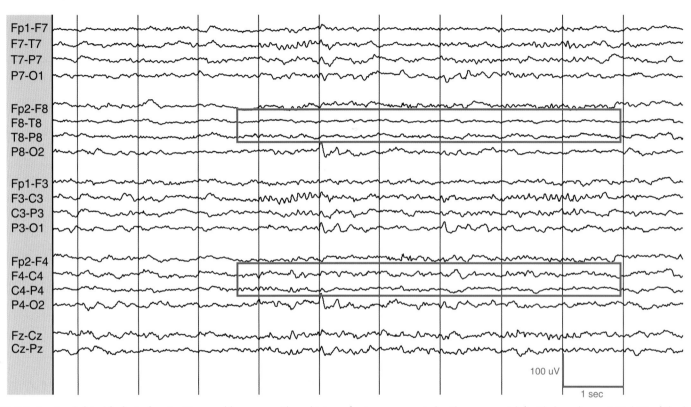

FIGURE 7.3 Acute right-sided stroke. An 83-year-old woman with no history of seizures presented with new-onset left-sided weakness. Initial CT of the head was negative for acute findings. EEG during sleep shows attenuation of fast frequencies and loss of sleep spindles over the right hemisphere *(boxes)*, concerning for an acute stroke. (Intervening fluid collection such as subdural hematoma can have similar findings, but this was ruled out by the CT head.) Repeat head CT the following day confirmed an acute right middle cerebral artery ischemic stroke.

For example, the usual EEG picture in cases of middle cerebral artery occlusion reveals reduction of fast frequencies and an irregular or polymorphic delta focus in the involved hemisphere, maximal in frontal, temporal, and parietal regions. In addition, the PDR is usually disrupted. During sleep, depression of sleep spindles and vertex waves on the side of the stroke may provide additional evidence of focal cerebral dysfunction.

When edema supervenes, the slowing may be more profound. Indeed, if the patient is lethargic, possibly due to midline intracranial shift, the opposite hemisphere will also demonstrate slowing and disorganization. Associated increased intracranial pressure or infarcts in the deep white matter may be accompanied by intermittent, frontally predominant generalized rhythmic delta activity (GRDA).

Occipital strokes present a different picture. Slowing over the posterior temporal and occipital regions may be evident, along with the ipsilateral reduction or destruction of the PDR (Fig. 7.4). Note that photic stimulation may evoke an asymmetric driving response, with depression over the involved side.

When the eyes open, the PDR attenuates in most normal controls. Unilateral failure of this attenuation can be caused by ipsilateral parietal and temporal lobe lesions. This can be an early and subtle sign of stroke or other lesion and is commonly known as Bancaud phenomenon.

Occlusion of the anterior cerebral artery usually results in frontal slowing, sometimes with frontal lateralized rhythmic delta activity (LRDA) or even frontally predominant GRDA. In such cases, the occipital rhythms are preserved.

Many strokes are subcortical, with sparing of the overlying cortex. Lacunar strokes involving the internal capsule or basal ganglia are common in patients with hypertension and are not always easy to differentiate clinically from those with cortical/subcortical involvement. Instead of demonstrating focal slowing, the record in these patients is usually normal. Alternatively, it may contain a mild diffuse abnormality, with or without lateralizing features.

Patients with clinically suspected transient ischemic attacks are often referred for an EEG. In these cases, the record is usually normal or nonfocal if obtained after resolution of the neurological findings. In some cases, however, intermittent focal slowing may be evident, suggesting that residual cerebral dysfunction is indeed present despite a normal neurological examination. If the EEG is obtained while the patient is symptomatic, appropriate focal slowing may be evident.

HEMORRHAGIC STROKE

Hemorrhagic strokes present a highly variable EEG picture, depending on the site of involvement, extent of the pathology, and the patient's state of awareness. A relatively small hemorrhage in the centrum semiovale likely results in a minor degree of lateralized slowing. On the other hand, basal ganglia hemorrhages with obtundation can demonstrate bilateral delta activity. Lateralization to the involved side may be seen, although in the face of depressed consciousness, asymmetry may not be evident. GRDA is common in such cases.

SUBDURAL HEMATOMA

The classic EEG finding in SDH is depression of cerebral activity over the involved hemisphere. This so-called insulation defect consists of reduced amplitude as compared with the opposite hemisphere. In addition, the PDR may be disrupted or even absent. If the collection is large, associated slowing may be evident. It should be emphasized that there is considerable variability in the EEG, and the classic finding of background depression is not always seen. If the SDH is small, there may be no obvious EEG findings.

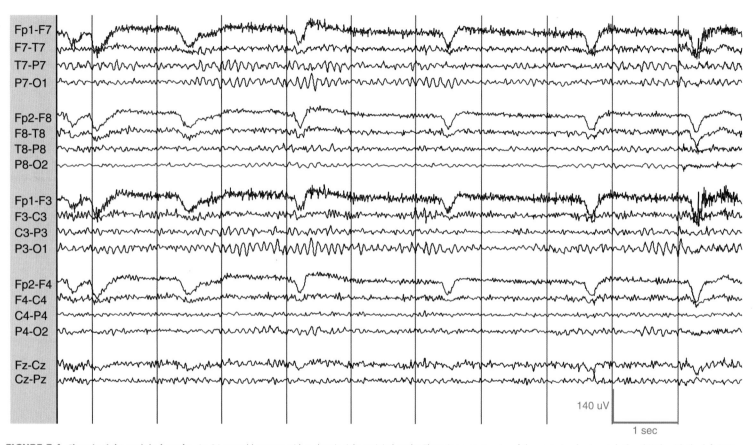

FIGURE 7.4 Chronic right occipital stroke. An 84-year-old woman with a chronic right occipital stroke. There is an asymmetry of the posterior dominant rhythm (PDR), with the left PDR being more than twice the amplitude of the right PDR. Higher amplitude on the right is commonly seen in normal subjects, and this is more than the allowable amplitude asymmetry.

Similarly, unilateral depression of cerebral activity can be seen in subdural hygromas and atrophic processes secondary to congenital brain damage. In addition, porencephaly leads to striking focal depression of the background that may present as an essentially isopotential (flat) picture.

METABOLIC DISORDERS

Clinically, metabolic disorders can result in a mildly altered mental status, personality changes, or even coma. The hallmark of a metabolic encephalopathy is diffuse slowing. In addition, the PDR is invariably disrupted, slowed, or absent. The slowing may be mild or profound, depending on the extent of the encephalopathy and the level of consciousness. The slowing is usually symmetric unless there is an underlying focal cerebral lesion unrelated to the metabolic disorder. In such cases, one may see focal and diffuse slowing. While recording, the technologist should attempt to arouse the patient. This may result in an increase in the background frequency, which is a demonstration of EEG reactivity.

In addition to diffuse slowing, frontally predominant GRDA may be recorded. Note that frontally predominant GRDA is a nonspecific finding and may also be seen in intoxications, increased intracranial pressure, and deep structural lesions.

An important feature of metabolic encephalopathies is generalized periodic discharges (GPDs), which can be with or without a triphasic morphology (Fig. 7.5). Classically, the initial deflection of a triphasic wave is negative (upgoing, fastest), the second deflection is positive (downgoing, tallest), and the third deflection is negative (upgoing, slowest). In addition, the classic triphasic wave demonstrates an anterior-posterior delay; that is, the frontal component leads the posterior component by 100 ms or so. GPDs with triphasic morphology are classically seen in hepatic encephalopathy but can be seen with uremia, sepsis, and electrolyte disturbances. However, biphasic generalized sharp waves, focal and multifocal epileptiform potentials, and focal and generalized seizures can be seen in toxic metabolic states.

It is not possible on visual inspection to delineate between GPDs secondary to a toxic metabolic cause and GPDs secondary to other causes. Both may have triphasic morphology. GPDs of any cause often increase with stimulation and improve with sleep. It is important to remember that GPDs faster than 2.5 Hz for greater than 10 seconds meet criteria for electrographic seizures (ESz).

CYCLIC ALTERNATING PATTERN OF ENCEPHALOPATHY (CAPE)

CAPE describes a background pattern spontaneously alternating between two phases, with each phase lasting at least 10 seconds and for at least six cycles in a relatively regular manner. One pattern often represents the more alert or stimulated pattern for the patient (Fig. 8.8). CAPE is observed in patients with encephalopathy of various etiologies and without normal sleep cycles on EEG. However, the clinical significance of CAPE has not been elucidated yet and requires further study.

Coma

In coma, the EEG can show a wide variety of patterns including but not limited to alpha coma, burst suppression, or even nonconvulsive status epilepticus (NCSE). The clinical examination can be identical for all of these patterns, and the approach to the patient and prognosis varies depending on the EEG findings and etiology of the coma.

Alpha coma

This is a distinct EEG constellation, usually resulting from widespread cerebral damage (as from anoxia). In this case, the rhythmic alpha characteristically appears most prominently in the frontal derivations but

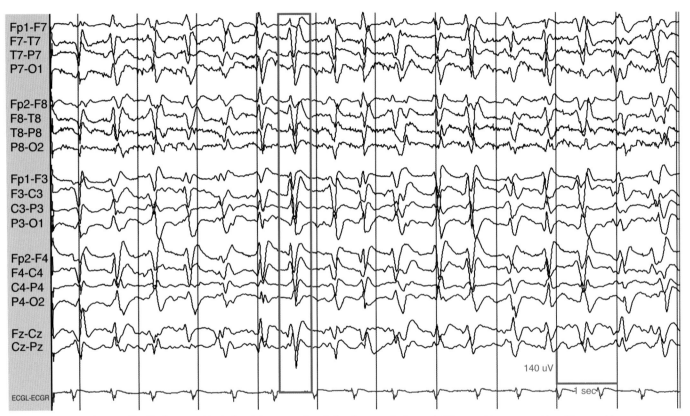

FIGURE 7.5 Generalized periodic discharges (GPDs), with a mostly triphasic morphology. A 66-year-old woman with a history of breast cancer presented with altered mental status. EEG shows continuous, generalized periodic sharp waves of mostly triphasic morphology, occurring at 2 Hz. An example of a triphasic wave with an anterior to posterior lag is seen in the *box*.

may be diffusely represented. There is no response to external stimuli or passive opening of the eyes. State change is absent. These findings usually imply a poor prognosis despite the lack of any diffuse slowing. If the alpha is more dominant posteriorly (as is seen in the normal population) and attenuates with alerting stimuli, the possibility of a patient in a locked-in state should be considered. Alpha coma is the best example of an EEG with severe dysfunction without any slowing.

Theta or delta coma

If the background shows predominantly delta or theta activity, the coma can be termed a delta/theta coma. This pattern is seen in a wide variety of etiologies, and the prognosis largely depends on the cause.

Spindle coma

In spindle coma, the EEG includes prominent spindlelike activity, similar to that seen in N2 sleep. It is typically seen with high mesencephalic lesions and portends a better outcome than alpha coma.

Beta coma

Beta coma is characterized by beta activity, sometimes frontally predominant. Beta coma is often the result of intoxication with barbiturates or benzodiazepines, and it generally portends a favorable outcome.

Burst suppression

The term burst suppression refers to a cycling of marked depression of cerebral activity (<10uV) and bursts of cerebral activity of variable amplitude, duration, and waveform (Figs. 4.5 and 7.6). The periods of suppression must occupy 50%–99% of the record to count as a burst suppression pattern. The bursts may be composed of multiphasic delta components, admixtures of various frequencies, or epileptiform activity

such as spikes or sharp waves, often with admixed slow components. The prototype of this phenomenon is found in patients receiving general anesthesia. It is thought that burst suppression results from suppression of cortical activity via γ-aminobutyric acid (GABA)-ergic mechanisms, with breakthrough EEG activity due to intact glutaminergic transmission. Under progressively deepening anesthesia, there are sequential EEG changes from normal sleep patterns, to diffuse delta waves, then burst-suppression, and finally isopotentiality. The burst suppression pattern is medically induced, often with anesthetics, in patients with refractory status epilepticus or other conditions in which it is desirable to lower metabolic demand of the brain.

Postcardiac arrest EEG. The EEG can play an important role in prognostication for people after cardiac arrest. The prognosis can only be discussed in patients who are off sedating medications and not hypothermic. The patterns considered *highly malignant* are (1) a suppressed background, (2) continuous GPDs with suppression between discharges, (3) burst suppression without epileptiform discharges (including identical bursts), and (4) burst suppression with superimposed discharges (including highly epileptiform bursts). These patterns all portend a poor outcome (Fig. 7.7). Notably, the *highly malignant* patterns have suppression (<10uV) as the common element. A *malignant* EEG pattern can be (1) periodic or rhythmic discharges +/– ESz, (2) discontinuous or low-voltage background, and (3) an unreactive EEG. Any two malignant patterns predict a poor outcome, whereas a single malignant pattern could have a good outcome. EEGs without the above features are considered benign and the outcome is likely to be good. The most common associated seizure post anoxic injury is myoclonus, and it is not yet known if treatment of this seizure type in this clinical circumstance improves the outcome.

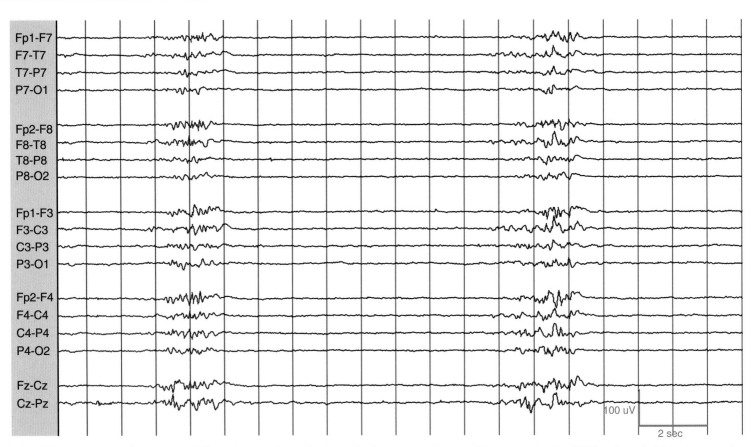

FIGURE 7.6 Burst-suppression pattern. A 74-year-old woman in a sedated coma for the treatment of nonconvulsive status epilepticus (NCSE) in the medical intensive care unit. The bursts consist of a mixture of theta and delta frequencies lasting 1–2 seconds, which alternate with periods of suppression lasting for 6–12 seconds.

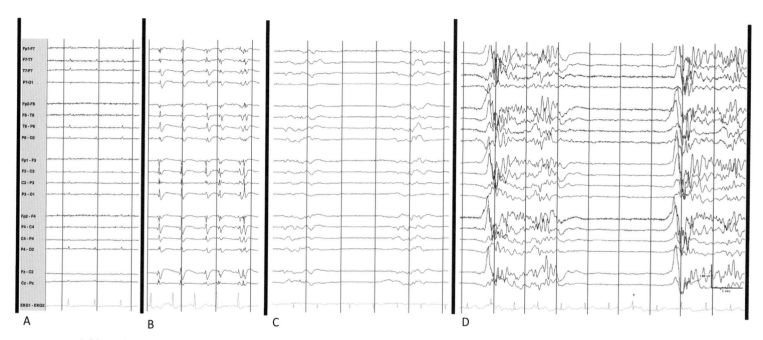

FIGURE 7.7 Highly malignant postanoxic EEG patterns. EEGs from four different patients status post cardiac arrest and off sedation show (A) diffuse suppression with low-amplitude EKG artifact, (B) generalized periodic discharges (GPDs) in a suppressed background, (C) burst suppression, and (D) burst suppression with identical highly epileptiform bursts. All patients died shortly after.

STATUS EPILEPTICUS

"If the possessing demon possesses him many times during the middle watch of the night, and at the time of his possession his hands and feet are cold, he is much darkened, keeps opening and shutting his mouth … It may go on for some time, but he will die."

From a tablet written in Babylon in 600–700 BCE

Status epilepticus, ongoing intermittent or continuous uncontrolled seizures, has long been recognized to pose severe danger to the individual in its grips. Several millennia after this quote was written on a cuneiform tablet in Babylon, status epilepticus still causes significant mortality and morbidity. The question becomes: at what point does a seizure become status? The average length of a generalized tonic-clonic (GTC) seizure is less than 2 minutes and the exact moment of irreversible neuronal injury is not known, *likely varying* between individuals. Furthermore, the risk of the seizure depends upon the seizure type. There are two critical time points in the conceptualization of status epilepticus, according to the International League Against Epilepsy (ILAE). The first, t_1, results from the failure of mechanisms responsible for seizure termination, and the second time point, t_2, is defined as the point after which there can be long-term consequences, including irreversible, long-term neuronal damage. On a practical level, t_1 is any seizure >5 minutes and the time to initiate treatment. T_2 is the time to consider intubation and a sedating medication. Every seizure type (tonic-clonic, tonic, clonic, myoclonic, absence, or focal) can become status epilepticus. For convulsive status epilepticus, t_2 is 30 minutes. For focal motor (i.e., epilepsia partialis continua [EPC]) and absence status, it is not clear if there is ever irreversible long-term damage and often, the goal in care is to manage without intubation.

Status epilepticus can elude diagnosis as people in focal status or even absence status may present with bizarre behavior and altered mentation. In addition, patients with lethargy, obtundation, or coma may well be having NCSE. NCSE can occur after convulsive status epilepticus or without any prior clinical seizures. Any individual who has had clinical seizures and is not back to baseline should be urgently connected to video-EEG (VEEG) as the distinction between a postictal state and ongoing seizure activity cannot be made clinically.

NCSE is especially common in critically ill patients and in fact, most seizures (about 75% on average in the literature) that occur in these patients are nonconvulsive and cannot be identified without an EEG. In any patient who is critically ill with a depressed level of consciousness, with or without known neurological problems, NCSE should be on the differential. It is particularly important as NCSE is a potentially treatable cause of obtundation and coma.

Unequivocal ESz are defined as (1) generalized or focal spike-wave discharges >2.5 Hz and >10 seconds (Fig. 7.8); or (2) clearly evolving discharges of any type >10 seconds (Fig. 7.9). An EEG pattern is said to evolve if there are at least two unequivocal sequential changes in frequency, morphology, or location. Electrographic status is defined as an ESz for >10 minutes or for more than 20% of any 60-minute period. A tonic-clonic seizure >5 minutes is considered electroclinical status epilepticus (ECSE).

When the EEG pattern does not meet the above criteria, it does not mean that it is not a seizure; it may or may not be. We know that at least 6 cm² of cortex needs to be involved to see seizures on surface electrodes. Intracranial EEG recordings, with electrodes directly on the surface of the brain or within the brain, can show focal seizures that are not seen on simultaneous surface extracranial electrodes.

As discussed in Chapter 4, certain electrographic features are more likely to be associated with seizures. For example, when periodic discharges (PDs) are associated with superimposed fast frequencies (+F), this pattern is considered more likely to be ictal than a pattern with PDs without +F. For EEG patterns in the gray zone, the term ictal-interictal continuum (IIC) is used. IIC is defined as (1) any PD or spike-and-wave or sharp-and-wave (SW) pattern >1 Hz but ≤2.5 Hz for greater than 10 seconds or (2) any PD or SW pattern ≥0.5 Hz and ≤1 Hz for greater than 10 seconds and has a + modifier or fluctuation, or (3) any lateralized

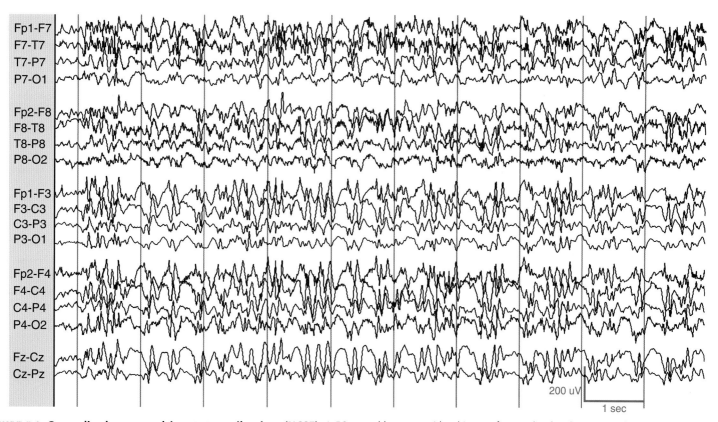

FIGURE 7.8 Generalized nonconvulsive status epilepticus (NCSE). A 56-year-old woman with a history of generalized epilepsy was admitted with altered mental status and no verbal output. EEG revealed nearly continuous generalized spike/polyspike/sharp and wave discharges at medium to high amplitude, fluctuating in frequencies up to 7 Hz, meeting the criteria for NCSE.

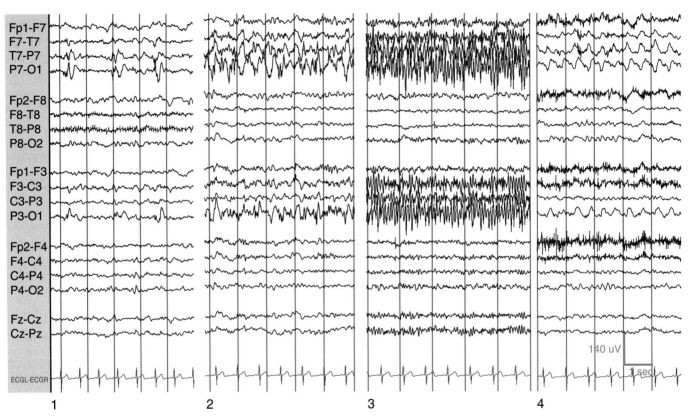

FIGURE 7.9 Focal status epilepticus. A 62-year-old man with a left parietal astrocytoma presents with altered mental status. Sequential EEG shows an evolving focal seizure. The seizure starts with left posterior periodic sharp waves and spikes (lateralized periodic discharges) *(1)*, which become faster in frequency *(2)*, with spread to other regions in the left hemisphere *(3)*. Postictally, there is rhythmic delta activity over the left posterior region (lateralized rhythmic delta activity) *(4)*. This seizure was occurring multiple times per hour without a return to his neurological baseline.

rhythmic delta activity (RDA) >1 Hz for at least 10 seconds and with a + modifier or fluctuation (Fig. 7.10). When the patient is obtunded with an IIC pattern, one may try administering a fast-acting antiseizure medication (ASM) and observe for clinical and electrographic improvements. If improvement occurs (particularly clinical improvement), the pattern should be considered NCSE. In critically ill patients, many findings can be missed from routine EEGs and it is recommended to do long-term EEG monitoring, especially if rhythmic or periodic patterns are present, because these are associated with increased risk of seizures.

Status epilepticus can occur in individuals who are medically ill, neurologically ill (brain tumor, stroke), and in patients with known epilepsy. In patients with epilepsy, status epilepticus typically happens because of medication noncompliance. Rarely, individuals will present with new-onset refractory status epilepticus (NORSE), the etiology of which is unclear (Fig. 7.11). These patients often have a mild febrile illness 1–2 weeks prior to the onset of unrelenting seizures that do not respond to standard ASMs. The etiology of NORSE is poorly understood but thought to be related to excess proinflammatory molecules. Status epilepticus in individuals who do not have known epilepsy should be evaluated for an underlying disorder like meningitis, encephalitis, sepsis, brain trauma, metabolic derangements, or stroke. In those cases, treatment of the status epilepticus is two-pronged: the individual is managed with ASMs (including anesthetic infusions if necessary) and aggressive treatment of the underlying process. For example, in an individual who presents in status with autoimmune limbic encephalitis, appropriate treatment includes ASMs and high-dose steroids. Treatment of status epilepticus is outlined in Appendix 2.

BRAIN DEATH

Brain death is essentially a clinical diagnosis. Under certain circumstances, an EEG might be ordered to confirm the diagnosis. The low-frequency filter should be set between 0.5 Hz and 1.5 Hz, and the high-frequency filter should be set at 70 Hz. For a brain death examination, the interelectrode impedance should be between 1000 and 10,000 Ohms. The EEG should be reviewed at a sensitivity of 2 µV/mm for at least 30 minutes, and a double-distance bipolar montage should be available to maximize the chances of detecting cerebral activity. Electrocerebral inactivity (ECI) is defined as the absence of any waves of cerebral origin. The record should not have activity that exceeds 2 µV unless that activity is a clear environmental artifact (e.g., an IV drip or cardiac artifact). In order to call this ECI consistent with brain death, reversible disturbances must be excluded (toxic-metabolic perturbations, hypothermia, or sedating medication).

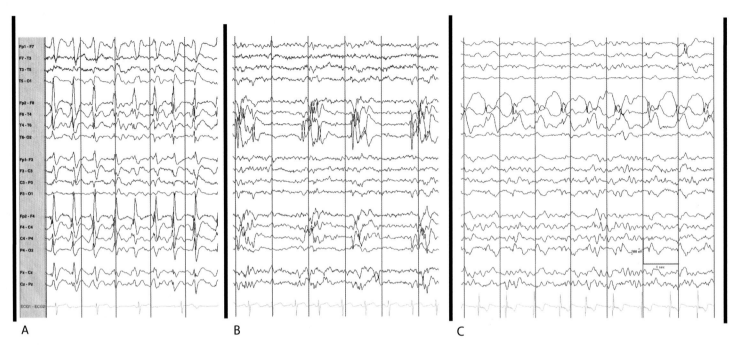

A   B   C

FIGURE 7.10 Ictal-interictal continuum (IIC). All patterns lasted >10 seconds. (A) Right frontally maximal 1.5–2 Hz lateralized periodic discharges in a 70-year-old woman with a right frontal hemorrhage. This pattern emerged after treatment of definite electrographic status epilepticus. (B) Right hemispheric (max P8) 0.5–1 Hz lateralized periodic discharges +F in an 85-year-old man with a right temporal parietal glioblastoma multiforme after admission for witnessed seizures. (C) Right temporal 1–1.5 Hz lateralized rhythmic delta activity + sharp waves (S) in a 7-year-old boy with developmental delay and a history of infantile spasms. Later in the same record, there were several hyperkinetic seizures, which were difficult to lateralize.

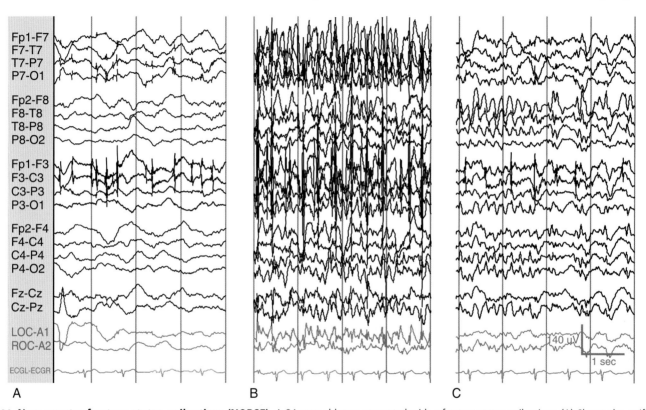

FIGURE 7.11 New-onset refractory status epilepticus (NORSE). A 31-year-old man presented with refractory status epilepticus. (A) Shows the artifact from ongoing left facial twitching. There is no electrographic right-sided seizure evident. (B) Hours later, he developed left facial twitching, which was more vigorous, and right hemisphere rhythmic activity can be discerned. (C) Ongoing right-sided electrographic seizure activity with a few left-sided facial twitches. Phenytoin, levetiracetam, midazolam, and ketamine failed to control his seizure activity, and he was placed in a pentobarbital coma.

Further reading

Hirsch, L.J., Fong, M.W.K., Leitinger, M., et al., 2021. American Clinical Neurophysiology Society's standardized critical care EEG terminology: 2021 Version. J. Clin. Neurophysiol 38, 1–29.

Trinka, E., Cock, H., Hesdorffer, D., et al., 2015. A definition and classification of status epilepticus—report of the ILAE task force on classification of status epilepticus. Epilepsia 56, 1515–1523.

Wieser, H.G., Schindler, K., Zumsteg, D., 2006. EEG in Creutzfeldt-Jakob disease. Clin. Neurophysiol. 117, 935–951.

Westhall, E., Rossetti, A.O., van Rootselaar, A.F., et al., 2016. Standardized EEG interpretation accurately predicts prognosis after cardiac arrest. Neurology 86, 1482–1490.

The goal of quantitative EEG (QEEG) is to provide the ICU clinicians with valuable information to make real-time treatment decisions as well as for the epileptologists to quickly glance through many hours of EEG and detect long-term trends. The American Clinical Neurophysiology Society (ACNS) recommends continuous EEG in the critically ill for a variety of conditions, including abnormal mental status after clinical seizures, acute supratentorial brain injury (like subarachnoid hemorrhage or traumatic brain injury) with an abnormal mental status, paroxysmal events that may or may not be seizures, and/or a routine EEG with periodic, rhythmic, or ictal patterns. These patients are at high risk for neurological deterioration because of ongoing nonconvulsive seizures, delayed cerebral ischemia, raised intracranial pressure, or CNS infection.

Ideal displays present information accurately with high sensitivity and specificity and allow clinicians to diagnose impending or occurring complications (for example, seizures or cerebral ischemia) and then visually see the effects of their interventions. The displays cannot be overly complex and yet they must be relevant. Patients with acute neurological issues are often in coma in the ICU, and we cannot rely on their neurological examinations to reflect underlying potential catastrophic changes in their brains. In this chapter, we will discuss each of the most salient elements separately and then discuss the challenges and the promise of synthesized real-time display.

THE ELEMENTS

QEEG in the ICU

For ongoing EEGs in the ICU, typically 10 seconds of real-time raw EEG data are displayed on the screen. Hours of raw signal are reviewed once or twice per day by a trained epileptologist. However, for patients with nonconvulsive status epilepticus or frequent seizures, more frequent checks are crucial in order to titrate medications and make treatment decisions. QEEG is an important supplement but not a replacement for raw EEG. For example, sensitivity for seizure detection using QEEG ranges from 50% to 70%, with frequent false-positives. When used alone, QEEG could cause unnecessary treatment of events that are not seizures and missed events that are seizures. We suggest that the raw EEG be reviewed by a trained epileptologist who can then identify for the ICU team the morphology of the specific seizure on QEEG.

QEEG can display multiple hours of compressed EEG data on a single screen. Overcompression of the signal (for example, including 24 hours of data on a single screen) will obscure events of interest. Typically, 2 hours of compressed EEG is ideal. In order for the data to be meaningful, it is not simply compressed, but different mathematical tools are used to transform the data and provide information in a visually digestible format. The visible panels and time scales are easy to adjust by the user so that the display can be customized for a specific patient.

Fast Fourier series transform (FFT) spectrogram

In an FFT, the EEG signal is broken up into component frequencies, usually between 0 and 20 Hz, with frequency on the y-axis. The x-axis is time, and again, this can be easily set by the user, but typically, 2 hours is displayed on a screen. At any moment in time, the abundance and amplitude of raw EEG at a given frequency are represented by a color power spectrum from blue (very little) to white (maximal). from blue (very little) to white (maximal). The signal is usually divided into two FFTs, one using all electrodes on the left hemisphere and one using all electrodes on the right hemisphere. For very focal events, the FFT can be displayed using fewer electrodes as input, for example, by quadrants (Figs. 8.1–8.8).

Rhythmicity spectrogram

The rhythmicity spectrogram is a proprietary mathematical computation (Persyst) in which the rhythmicity of the EEG at four frequency bands from 1 to 25 Hz is displayed using a color scale, with deep blue being most rhythmic and pale yellow being not rhythmic. Each spectrogram can be configured by hemisphere, by channel, or by quadrant, depending on the needs (Figs. 8.1, 8.5, 8.7, and 8.8). For example, a focal left frontal seizure may be undetectable looking at the left hemisphere electrodes together but very apparent if one looks at only the left anterior quadrant.

Amplitude EEG (aEEG)

This display outputs the EEG signal amplitude (from peak to peak) as a function of time. The right hemisphere is displayed with a red line and the left hemisphere is displayed with a blue line. When the hemispheres are symmetric in amplitude, the color becomes fuchsia. Seizures nearly always cause a change in aEEG and often a divergence between the hemispheres (Figs. 8.3, 8.4, and 8.5).

Asymmetry index/spectrogram

Asymmetry displays a comparison of the power of the EEG in homologous right and left electrodes at each frequency. The color scale for this spectrogram is simply red for when the right has increased power compared to the left and blue for when the left is greater than the right. The asymmetry spectrogram can show asymmetry at the patient's baseline as well as changes over time which can occur with seizures, evolving infarcts, and state changes (Figs. 8.4, 8.7, and 8.8).

Alpha-delta ratios

The alpha-delta ratio is essentially a measurement of the degree of slowing in the EEG. The higher the ratio, the faster the EEG. Decreasing alpha-delta ratio can be a marker of vasospasm and impending cerebral ischemia. When cerebral blood flow (CBF) decreases to below normal, the first change in the EEG is the loss of faster frequencies; as CBF becomes more compromised, there is an increase in slower frequencies. The EEG change occurs within seconds of the change in the CBF. In both cases, there is a decrease in the alpha-delta ratio. The raw EEG is not ideal for detecting these changes as subtle changes over time are easy to miss (Fig. 8.6).

Suppression index

This trend displays the percentage of EEG that is suppressed as a function of time. The higher the level of suppression, the higher the line of the trend will be (Figs. 8.4 and 8.5).

Versus baseline control spectrogram

This panel takes the patient's own baseline EEG and demonstrates changes from that baseline. Specifically, the power in each frequency is compared to the empiric null using the number of standard deviations (z-score) represented by color (green to blue: negative z-score; green to red: positive z-score) (Fig. 8.8)

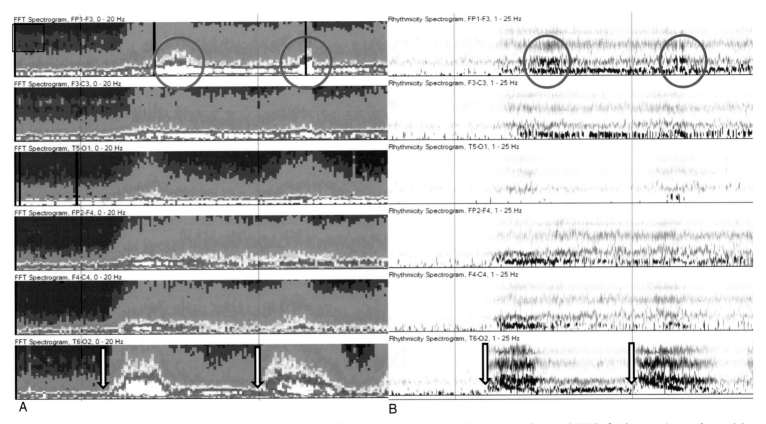

FIGURE 8.1 The FFT spectrogram (A) and the rhythmicity spectrogram (B) of a patient in nonconvulsive status epilepticus (NCSE) of right posterior quadrant origin; 20 minutes of compressed data shown. Seizure onsets are best seen in the right posterior quadrant (T8-02) in both panels. The seizure is seen to spread from the right posterior quadrant *(arrows)* to the left anterior quadrant *(circles)*.

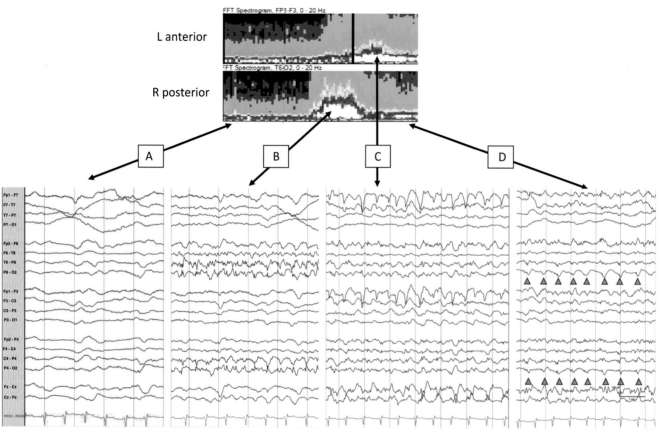

FIGURE 8.2 The FFT for the left anterior *(top)* and right posterior *(bottom)* regions shown for the first seizure in Fig. 8.1. Raw EEG before the seizure shows diffuse slowing (A); then right posterior seizure (B); then seizure spread to the left anterior region (C), followed by subtle right posterior lateralized periodic discharges (LPDs) *(Blue triangles)* (D).

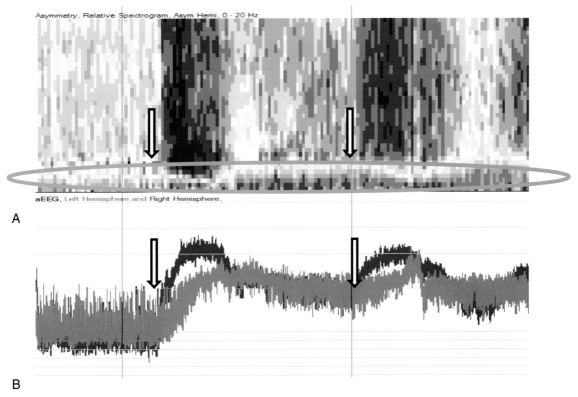

FIGURE 8.3 The relative asymmetry spectrogram (A) and the amplitude EEG (aEEG) (B) during the same two seizures *(arrows)* as shown in Fig. 8.1. Blue is the left hemisphere and red is the right hemisphere. At the seizure onset, there is an abrupt increase in power on the right in frequencies greater than the delta range. This continues even after the seizure ends and corresponds to subtle faster frequencies throughout the right hemisphere. During seizures, the amplitude of the EEG increases in both hemispheres but more so on the right.

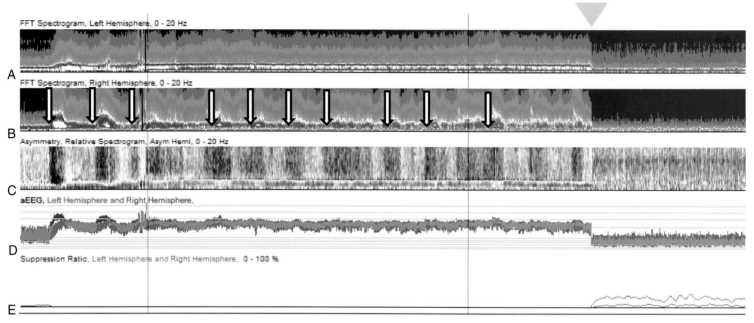

FIGURE 8.4 Two hours of compressed data from the same patient. Discrete seizures *(arrows)* seen best in the right hemisphere FFT spectrogram (B) become more subtle. With infusion of fosphenytoin *(yellow caret)*, there is abrupt cessation of seizures and the FFT spectrograms (A, B) show a decrease in power at all frequency bands. At this moment, the asymmetry spectrogram (C) shows more power on the left compared with the right. The amplitude EEG (aEEG) (D) shows an abrupt drop in amplitude, and the suppression spectrogram (E) shows that both sides become suppressed, with the right being more suppressed than the left.

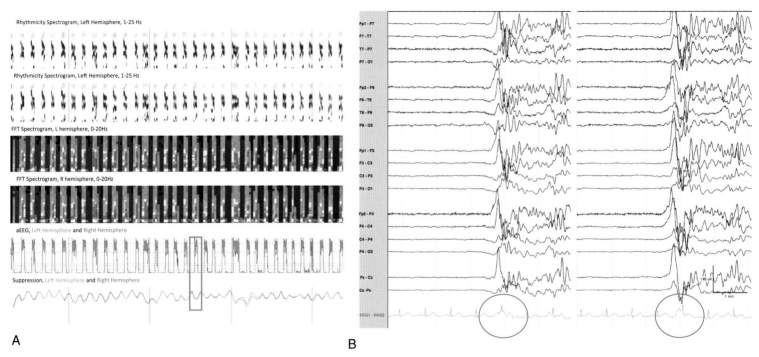

A

B

FIGURE 8.5 Identical highly epileptiform burst suppression. A 65-year-old man after cardiac arrest on no sedation. (A) Twenty minutes of compressed EEG. Rhythmicity spectrogram shows bands of rhythmic bursts in alpha and beta frequencies. Amplitude EEG (aEEG) reflects a symmetric increase in amplitude with each burst as the suppression ratio decreases *(green box)*. (B) Raw EEG confirms symmetric burst suppression pattern with identical highly epileptiform bursts. Slight artifact in the EKG lead at the start of the burst is caused by very subtle myoclonus *(red oval)*, making the diagnosis of myoclonic status epilepticus.

Alpha-Delta Ratios

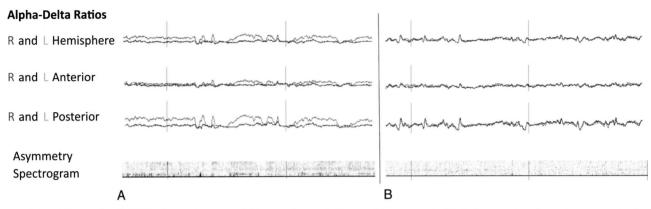

R and L Hemisphere

R and L Anterior

R and L Posterior

Asymmetry
Spectrogram

A   B

FIGURE 8.6 **Alpha-delta ratios (ADRs) after subarachnoid hemorrhage**. A 47-year-old woman admitted after a ruptured anterior communicating artery aneurysm. (A) Asymmetric ADRs seen on posthemorrhage day 5 with decreased right (red) ADRs, most marked posteriorly. Asymmetry spectrogram shows increased power in the slower frequencies on the right (red). The patient was awake and without focal neurological signs. Left upper extremity pronator drift developed on day 6. The patient was taken for an angiogram, where right multifocal vasospasm was confirmed and treated with intraarterial verapamil. On day 10 (B), the ADRs were symmetric and the patient was neurologically intact.

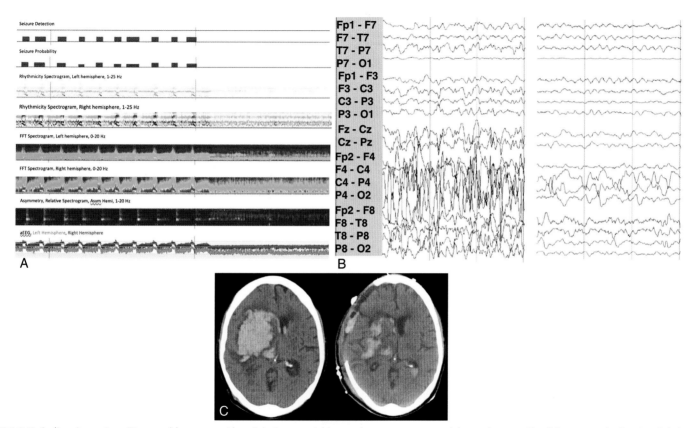

FIGURE 8.7 Cyclic seizures in a 58-year-old woman with a right intracranial hemorrhage status post a right craniectomy. The 6-hour quantitative EEG (A) shows cyclic right hemispheric seizures with increased rhythmicity, power, and amplitude (right > left) during each of the seizures. Seizures cease with IV lacosamide. Raw EEG (B) shows high-amplitude, chaotic-appearing right seizure activity different from the patient's background, and (C) demonstrates the hemorrhage pre and post craniectomy on a head CT scan..

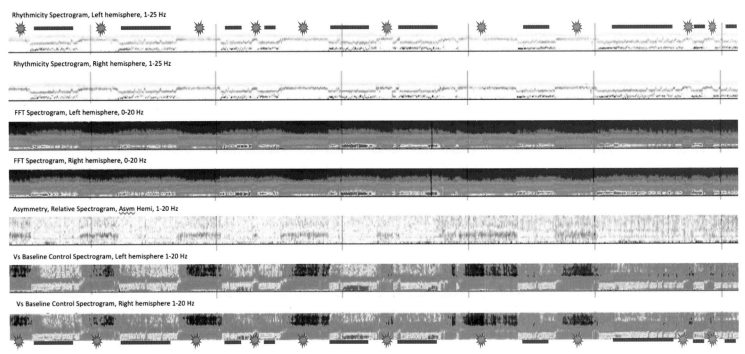

A

FIGURE 8.8 Cyclic alternating pattern of encephalopathy (CAPE) in a 58-year-old man who presented with a high-grade subarachnoid hemorrhage and hydrocephalus. (A) Twelve hours of compressed data.

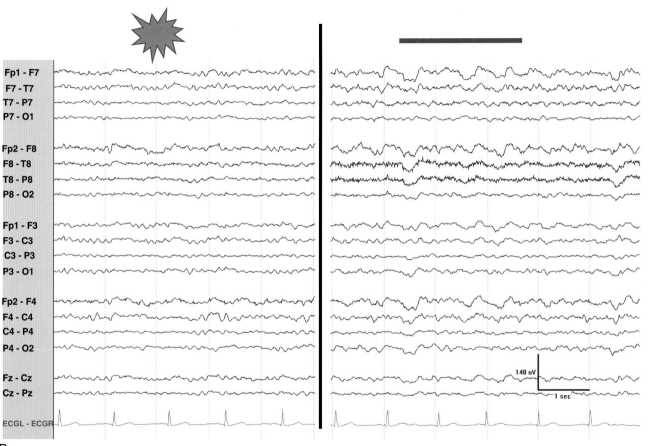

B

FIGURE 8.8 cont'd (B) Raw EEG. One pattern has increased alpha *(star)* and the second pattern is more in the delta/theta range *(dark line)*. Versus baseline control spectrogram (A) displays this alternating pattern more distinctly, comparing the power in each frequency with the empirical null using the number of standard deviations (z-score) represented by color (green to blue: negative z-score; green to red: positive z-score).

This spectrogram is useful when determining the presence of reactivity and state change.

Further reading

Hirsch, L.J., et al., 2021. American Clinical Neurophysiology Society's standardized critical care EEG terminology: 2021 Version. J. Clin. Neurophysiol 38 (1), 1–29.

Hirsch, L.J., Brenner, R.P., 2010. Atlas of EEG in Critical Care, first ed. Wiley, Chichester.

Kaleem, S., Swisher, C.B., 2022. Utility of quantitative EEG for seizure detection in adults. J. Clin. Neurophysiol 39 (3), 184–194.

Suzette, M.L., Hiba, A.H., 2018. Handbook of ICU EEG Monitoring, second ed. Demos Medical, New York.

The EEG: Tips on indications, reading, and reporting   9

INDICATIONS

Routine EEG

- Assessment of patients with suspected seizures, epilepsy, or transient events. If normal, depending on the level of suspicion, a repeat routine EEG, a sleep-deprived study, or a long-term EEG may be indicated.
- Follow up assessment after the introduction of antiseizure medications (ASMs) in patients with epilepsy.
- Follow up assessment after the cessation of ASMs.
- Altered mental status of unknown cause. If unrevealing, then prolonged EEG monitoring may be needed.
- Confirmation of brain death.
- Evaluation of prognosis in coma.

Inpatient VEEG monitoring

- Characterization of seizures in a person with known epilepsy who is undergoing a presurgical evaluation.
- Determination of seizure frequency when undetected seizures are suspected. For example, if a patient with known epilepsy is having worsening memory problems, there may be subclinical seizures affecting cognition.

- Distinguishing among epileptic or psychogenic nonepileptic seizures (PNES) and other seizure mimics.
- Changing medications in a controlled and safe environment.
- Management of ongoing seizures or status epilepticus.
- Ongoing monitoring in patients with lethargy, obtundation, and coma to ascertain if the altered level of consciousness is caused by ongoing seizures.
- Surveillance for delayed cerebral ischemia with raw and quantitative EEG in patients with subarachnoid hemorrhage due to aneurysmal rupture.

If seizure characterization is desired, various provocation techniques are carried out during the study, including hyperventilation, photic stimulation, and sleep deprivation.

Ambulatory EEG (AEEG) monitoring

This long-term monitoring technique has the attraction of sending the patient home with a small, portable EEG amplifier, with or without a camera. Typically, the patient carries out normal activities and keeps a diary of any events that occur. Recording may be carried out for days. Family members or friends can aid in the note keeping as the patient may be unaware of events. Indications are more constricted than the indications for in-patient video-EEG (VEEG) as it is not appropriate to stop medications to capture seizures or (obviously) to manage status epilepticus at home.

HOW TO LOOK AT THE RECORD

The beginner electroencephalographer is faced with an endless array of wiggly lines, and the meaning behind those lines can be elusive. The task of discerning clinically relevant information seems, at first, impossible. Like learning to interpret musical notes or to read in a foreign language, the secret to success is practice and exposure. In addition, the electroencephalographer should develop an armature, or a systematic underlying structure, on which the information in each EEG can be reported. This report provides useful information to the clinician, with the goal of ultimately improving the quality of life of our patients.

In order to interpret the record properly, one must have clearly in mind the elements of a normal EEG. This establishes a template against which all deviations are to be compared. It is useful to analyze carefully the first few interpretable epochs with the intention of creating a basic scaffold onto which further details will be added later. One may begin to ascertain the background, including systematic thought to the continuity, symmetry, organization, and reactivity of the record. Is there a reactive posterior dominant rhythm (PDR)? If there is no PDR, is the record reactive to stimulation? Technicians should give nail bed pressure and passively open and close the eyes of any patient who does not fully alert with voice or a gentle shake. Abnormalities may be glaring, as in a burst suppression pattern, or one may appreciate a hint of focality, paroxysmal activity, or a possible asymmetry of background activity. If the patient is awake at the onset of the EEG, it is good to repeat this careful analysis in the first epoch of sleep. The symmetry and presence of sleep transients (sleep spindles, vertex waves, K-complexes, and positive occipital sharp transients of sleep [POSTs]) should be noted as well as the presence of sleep stages. N3 sleep (slow wave sleep) is not often seen in a routine EEG or in hospitalized patients. N2 sleep is a particularly fruitful time for the appearance of epileptiform discharges, if present.

After the first few minutes of the EEG are scrutinized, the experienced electroencephalographer will often begin to speed through pages at a rapid rate. With wiggly lines racing by, the electroencephalographer is looking with a relaxed and alert gaze at the whole screen, perhaps looking softly from the left-sided electrodes to the right-sided electrodes. This is somewhat akin to what we feel when we drive a car; we are alert, we are looking ahead, and we are ready to respond to anything unusual. When something does stand out from the background, the electroencephalographer will pause and focus. Perhaps the element that stood out from the background looks like a possible sharp wave. The wave should be scrutinized in different montages. First, the longitudinal bipolar montage; is there a phase reversal? If so, at what electrode(s)? Is there an aftergoing slow wave? Once this has been established, the wave should be examined in a referential montage, with the hypothesis that the electrode with the phase reversal will have the highest amplitude in a reference montage (see Chapter 1). If the abnormality appears maximally in either the occipital or frontopolar electrodes, a circumferential montage should be used as phase reversals will not be apparent on the longitudinal bipolar montage (because of the end-of-chain effect). Many things will catch the novice's eye (e.g., muscle artifacts and wicket spikes). Before an element is called epileptiform, it must stand up to scrutiny. If there are abundant epileptiform potentials on one side, it is often useful to reread the record, with focus and attention on the quieter hemisphere to make sure that sharp waves and spikes are not missed.

The electroencephalographer will stop for a seizure. In this case, the video is examined and then the EEG is scrutinized in a very detailed manner. The semiology of the patient should be described in detail as semiology can help clinicians lateralize and even localize seizures. Then we seek to identify the exact electrographic onset, so it is necessary to backtrack from the obvious onset to see if there is perhaps a more subtle onset that was missed.

If there is a flurry of movement artifact, the electroencephalographer should pause and look at the video (if present). EEGs are often ordered for an evaluation of an unusual movement, and any strange movements should be commented on in the report.

The EEG may be annotated with notes of clinical events reported by the patient, a family member, or the nursing staff. These events should be analyzed in detail. As mentioned in Chapter 5, the diagnosis often depends on the video as an event without EEG change can either be a surface-negative seizure or a seizure mimic like PNES. The semiology of the event can in many cases clarify the diagnosis. For all events, the EKG strip should be reviewed and any EKG correlates should be reported on.

ELEMENTS OF THE REPORT

Guidelines provided by the American Clinical Neurophysiology Society (ACNS) should be followed so that the nomenclature used in the EEG report is standardized (Table 4.1). After all, what one neurologist means by "frequent" may be different from what the next neurologist means by "frequent." Table 9.1 outlines a standard order for an EEG report.

Table 9.1 The EEG report	
History	The patient's name, date of birth, medical record number, location, date of recording, and total recording time should appear at the top of the report. In addition, the reason for the EEG request and any medications that affect the central nervous system are reported in this section. For EMU and intracranial reports, the patient's typical seizures should be described.
Technical description	The software, the number of electrodes used, the type of EEG (routine, sleep-deprived, in patient, long-term, intracranial, etc.), and the presence or absence of video should be noted. Any spike or event detection programs used should be noted. If the recording is intracranial, the electrode array should be described and a diagram should be included.
EEG description	If the study is a multiday study, this section of the report should be repeated for each day. Medication changes should be noted for each day.
Background	
Organization	Organization should be described as good, fair, or poor. Absence or presence of a PDR and a normal A-P gradient is noted. Features of organization of neonates and children are age specific (Chapter 3).
Symmetry/frequency	A description of the predominant frequencies is recorded. A comparison of frequency and amplitude is made between the left and right sides. Slowing, if present, is described in terms of location (generalized/focal), prevalence, and morphology (polymorphic/monomorphic). RDA is placed in the section with epileptiform abnormalities as it can be a marker of cortical hyperexcitability. Breach artifacts (higher amplitude with increased frequency due to skull defects) are noted. Focal and generalized attenuation is noted.

(Continued)

Table 9.1 The EEG report—cont'd

Sleep/state change	Note the absence or presence of state change. If state change is present, note if there are normal sleep transients. CAPE, if present, should be described. Note: if there is state change, the EEG is considered reactive.
Reactivity	In healthy patients, this is typically easy to identify—when the eyes are closed in a relaxed awake state, the PDR emerges. In comatose patients, it is not as easy to determine and one must rely on the technician. The technician typically opens and closes a patient's eyes. In catatonic patients who do not seem to react, passive eye opening and closure will bring out a PDR. In comatose patients, the technician should also administer noxious stimulation. Reactivity refers to a change in the brain waves, not the appearance of eye blinks or muscle artifact. If only SIRPIDs are present, it should be reported as reactive, SIRPIDs only. If reactivity lasts for < 60 seconds, the EEG is reactive without state change.
Continuity	Specify if the background is continuous, nearly continuous, discontinuous, or in a burst suppression/attenuation pattern. Duration of bursts and interburst intervals are noted. Morphology of bursts is described.
Activation procedures	Responses to photic stimulation and hyperventilation are described here.
Interictal epileptiform features	
Interictal epileptiform discharges, rhythmic or periodic patterns	List spikes, sharp waves, PDs, and RDA (both generalized and lateralized) in this section. Prevalence, frequency (cycles per second), location, morphology, duration, and presence in various states (sleep/wake/drowsiness) should be noted. Specify SIRPIDs, if present, and type of stimuli. *Example*: 1. Rare 3 Hz frontally predominant generalized spike and wave discharges of very brief duration, present in sleep 2. Abundant right parietal (P4) spikes, predominantly in wakefulness.
Seizures and events	
Seizures and events	The time and duration of the event, clinical description, and EEG findings appear under this heading. In addition, if someone is in electrographic status, a brief picture of the overall neurological state is placed here (e.g., "*The patient was lethargic on this day, rousable with noxious stimuli but unable to follow commands*"). For discrete events, describe the clinical and electrographic findings. *Example*: **Clinical:** Conitnuous 1 Hz right hand clonic movements with supination are present. These persist in sleep and are not suppressible during examination. **Electrographic:** There is no EEG correlate for the clinical finding.

Table 9.1 The EEG report—cont'd

Conclusion

Impression	List in summary the essential findings. We recommend sticking to the order of background first, then epileptiform abnormalities, and then seizures and events.
	Example: This is an abnormal EEG, demonstrating:
	1. Frequent left polymorphic delta frontotemporal slowing.
	2. Abundant left anterior temporal spikes (T7) in wakefulness and sleep.
	3. A single brief FIAS with subtle behavioral arrest of left anterior temporal origin.
Clinical correlation	This final section is perhaps the most important aspect of the report and represents the final translation of the EEG findings. If the findings support a diagnosis of left temporal lobe epilepsy, say it here. If the findings are consistent with a metabolic disorder or a structural lesion, then so indicate. If the findings are nonspecific, then list a succinct differential. In this section of the report, slowing, either focal or generalized, is often referred to as cerebral dysfunction, whereas spikes, sharp waves, PDs, LRDA and BIRDs are referred to as epileptiform potentials, cortical hyperexcitability, or cortical irritability.

A-P gradient, Anterior to posterior gradient; *CAPE*, cycle pattern of encephalopathy; *EMU*, epilepsy monitoring unit; *EPC*, epilepsia partialis continua; *FIAS*, focal impaired awareness seizure; *LRDA*, lateralized rhythmic delta activity; *BIRDs*, Brief potentially ictal rhythmic discharges; *PDs*, periodic discharges; *PDR*, posterior dominant rhythm; *RDA*, rhythmic delta activity; *SIRPIDs*, stimulation-induced rhythmic, periodic, or ictal discharges.

Further reading

American Clinical Neurophysiology Society Guidelines. www.acns.org.

American Clinical Neurophysiology Society Guidelines and Consensus Statements, Guideline 7: Guidelines for EEG reporting. J. Clin. Neurophysiol. 33 (4), 328–332.

American Clinical Neurophysiology Society Guidelines and Consensus Statements, 2008. Guideline 12: Guidelines for long-term monitoring for epilepsy. J. Clin. Neurophysiol. 25 (3), 170–180.

Kellaway, P., 2003. Orderly approach to visual analysis: elements of the normal EEG and their characteristics in children and adults. In: Ebersole, J.S., Pedley, T.A. (Eds.), Current Practice of Clinical Electroencephalography. Lippincott Williams & Wilkins, Philadelphia, pp. 100–159.

Influence of common drugs on the EEG and on seizure threshold

Many common medications have effects on the brain and thus on the EEG. Although these effects are not specific, it is important for our readers to be familiar with them in order to avoid an erroneous diagnosis of intrinsic brain pathology.

Antidepressants

Tricyclic antidepressants such as imipramine, amitriptyline, doxepin, desipramine, and nortriptyline usually increase the amount of beta activity, as well as theta activity in the record. The frequency of the posterior dominant rhythm (PDR) is sometimes decreased. Paroxysmal slow waves or even spikes may be seen. Acute intoxication may produce widespread, poorly reactive alpha-range activity and spikes. Absence status can be seen with tricyclic antidepressants.

The proconvulsant properties of antidepressants have been reported, but mostly anecdotally and from high dosages/overdoses. Lowered seizure thresholds are seen with bupropion (typically in doses of 450 mg a day or higher) and clomipramine. In people with epilepsy, there is a decreased incidence of seizures with other antidepressants, including several tricyclic antidepressants, selective serotonin reuptake inhibitors (SSRIs), serotonin-noradrenaline reuptake inhibitors, and the α2-antagonist mirtazapine. This may be due to the bidirectional relationship between psychiatric disorders and epilepsy. There are no definite effects on the EEG of the newer antidepressants.

SSRIs and other antidepressants can cause serotonin syndrome with mental status changes, autonomic instability, myoclonus, and tremor. The EEG in serotonin syndrome can show diffuse slowing, spikes, and generalized periodic discharges with a triphasic morphology.

With the exception of trazodone, nearly all antidepressants have been noted to decrease REM sleep with variable effects on N1, N2 and slow wave sleep.

Antimicrobial agents

β-Lactam antibiotics, specifically penicillin, the cephalosporins, and the carbapenems, are well-known to be proconvulsant, causing an altered mental status, jerks, generalized seizures, and even status epilepticus. The β-lactam ring can bind to the gamma-aminobutyric acid (GABA) receptor making GABA a less effective inhibitory neurotransmitter. For all of these agents, risk factors in the development of seizures include high doses, renal failure, and meningitis. Of all of these agents, imipenem, a carbapenem, is the worst culprit, causing seizures in approximately one-third of patients with meningitis. The EEG with β-lactam-induced encephalopathy is usually slow with generalized epileptiform potentials, at times with a triphasic morphology. Amoxicillin has been seen to induce spikes and polyspikes. Isoniazid and the fluoroquinolones are also known to lower the seizure threshold. Neurotoxic effects of quinolones include seizures, myoclonus, and encephalopathy. Diffuse slowing can be seen in patients with delirium from fluroquinolone usage. Among quinolones, the new quinolone derivatives or gyrase inhibitors (e.g., levofloxacin and moxifloxacin) are the ones most often associated with neurotoxic side effects, which are hypothesized to be from the activation of N-methyl-D-aspartate (NMDA) receptors and inhibition of GABA-A receptors.

Antiseizure medications

Phenytoin, unlike barbiturates and benzodiazepines, does not produce prominent beta activity. Rather, it tends to cause an increase in the degree of diffuse slow waves with increase of theta/delta frequencies and decrease of alpha frequencies. With chronic use there is usually a decline in the frequency of the PDR. At toxic levels, diffuse irregular delta activity may be recorded along with paroxysmal rhythmic delta activity.

Carbamazepine and oxcarbazepine usually have little effect on the EEG at therapeutic levels. An increase in diffuse slowing may occur. Epileptiform activity is usually not materially altered, although an increase in focal spikes has been reported. Rarely, generalized epileptiform potentials develop. Phenytoin, carbamazepine, oxcarbazepine, gabapentin, pregabalin and vigabatrin can worsen generalized epileptiform potentials and exacerbate absence and myoclonic seizures in people with generalized epilepsy.

Valproic acid at therapeutic levels produces little or no change in the EEG background. Its principal effect is a reduction in generalized epileptiform discharges, particularly 3 Hz generalized spike and wave discharges. At toxic levels, valproate may produce an encephalopathy characterized by lethargy with a recording dominated by diffuse delta waves. Furthermore, at high levels associated with hyperammonemic encephalopathy, triphasic waves can be seen arising from an abnormal background consisting of delta and theta activity.

Lamotrigine decreases the frequency of interictal spikes and sharp waves and is not associated with either increased beta activity or increased slowing. Lamotrigine can worsen (or ameliorate) myoclonic seizures and is notable for having minimal cognitive side effects. Levetiracetam decreases interictal epileptiform potentials typically without other effects on the EEG. It does not appear to slow the EEG background frequency. Lacosamide may also decrease the number of interictal spikes. Ethosuximide decreases generalized spike and wave and absence seizures. Topiramate may increase diffuse slowing with increased theta/delta frequencies and less alpha and beta frequencies. Zonisamide does not seem to influence the EEG.

As of this writing, there are a multitude of other antiseizure medications (ASMs) whose effects on the EEG are either minor and/or not fully investigated.

Barbiturates

Barbiturates produce an increase in the amount and amplitude of beta activity. The beta may reach high amplitudes and, although diffuse, is often most prominent in the frontal regions. As the blood level of the barbiturate rises, slower activity begins to invade the recording along with slowing of the PDR. Barbiturate intoxication leads to changes similar to those associated with general anesthesia. Diffuse, unreactive delta activity may be recorded, while beta activity disappears. Later stages lead to burst suppression and ultimately an isopotential or flat record. Abrupt withdrawal after long-term treatment may lead to asynchronous slowing along with generalized epileptiform activity and bursts of spikes and polyspikes.

Benzodiazepines

Like barbiturates, benzodiazepines produce prominent beta activity. Even after the last dose of one of these drugs, excessive beta may persist for some days. Some diffuse theta range slowing may be seen along with attenuation of the PDR. Paroxysmal synchronous slowing may be seen after long-term use. Effects of toxic doses are similar to those produced by other CNS depressants and correlate with the degree of mental status depression. Benzodiazepines have been shown to decrease the amount of N1 sleep (which can be helpful in people who suffer from insomnia) and decrease slow wave sleep.

Carbidopa/Levodopa

Pyridoxine deficiency (B6) is a known cause of intractable seizures in neonates and children. B6 deficiency causes epilepsy by decreasing production of GABA in the brain. However, in adults, recent cases of B6 deficiency in patients with Parkinson's Disease on Carbidopa/ Levodopa have been reported. B6 is a cofactor for the metabolism of levodopa into dopamine and can be depleted by excessive amounts of levodopa particularly in the setting of poor nutritional intake or weight loss. In these cases, the EEG can show diffuse slowing, focal or generalized epileptiform potentials as well as electrographic seizures that tend to be refractory to ASM but respond to B6 supplementation.

CNS toxins

There are a great number of agents that are toxic to the CNS and can cause acute, subacute, or chronic neurological symptoms. These include but are not limited to toxicity with lead, mercury, methyl alcohol, carbon monoxide, and organophosphate poisoning. The EEG findings are not specific for any one culprit and can include diffuse slowing and generalized epileptiform abnormalities. Focal epileptiform discharges have been reported as well.

Ethanol

Chronic alcoholics often have an EEG which is low in amplitude. In the first 48 hours of alcohol withdrawal syndrome, the EEG may be low in amplitude with generalized spikes or even lateralized periodic discharges (LPDs). Seizures and even status epilepticus are well known complications of alcohol withdrawal, particularly 6–48 hours after alcohol cessation. Alcohol withdrawal seizures are treated in the short term, usually with benzodiazepines, but other ASMs appear to be effective and safe. If epileptiform features persist after the period of acute withdrawal, the clinician should consider the possibility of nonalcohol-related seizures as well. Outside of alcohol withdrawal, people with chronic alcohol use disorder have a three-fold increased risk of developing epilepsy compared with the general population. While this is not fully understood, increased head trauma, cardiovascular disease, kindling with alcohol withdrawal seizures, and/or general poor nutrition and health are thought to contribute to the overall risk. Patients with epilepsy are advised to minimize or abstain from alcohol, as a seizure can follow even a single night of moderate to heavy drinking. Abrupt withdrawal of alcohol can induce bursts of spikes and polyspikes.

Lithium

Lithium may lead to diverse and prominent changes in the EEG. Although there is some correlation between the blood level of lithium and electrographic changes, there is considerable variability. One may see slowing of the PDR along with an increase in diffuse slowing. Intermittent rhythmic delta waves, most prominent in the frontal or occipital regions, may appear, and triphasic waves have been described. With lithium intoxication, EEG abnormalities are usually marked and include considerable diffuse slow waves, triphasic waves, and multifocal epileptiform discharges. These findings may linger for days after clinical manifestations of intoxication have resolved.

Marijuana

Smoking marijuana produces no visible changes in the EEG. Cannabidiol (CBD) appears to decrease the frequency of interictal epileptiform discharges. It does not appear to affect the background frequency. Epidiolex is an FDA approved CBD and prescribed to treat seizures in persons with Dravet syndrome, Lennox–Gastaut syndrome (LGS), or tuberous sclerosis complex.

Neuroleptics

Typical neuroleptics (e.g., phenothiazines) at therapeutic doses cause slowing of the PDR along with diffuse slow waves. They may also activate generalized delta activity and sharp waves. In patients with epilepsy, phenothiazines may increase seizure frequency, particularly at high or toxic doses.

The atypical neuroleptic, clozapine, produces an increase in diffuse slowing. Chronic use may lead to paroxysmal slowing with spikes or sharp waves. Of the antipsychotics, clozapine has been noted to be the most associated with epileptiform abnormalities, with some studies showing 47%–67% of patients with EEG abnormalities. More than other neuroleptics, clozapine lowers the seizure threshold and has been reported to cause generalized tonic clonic (GTC) seizures and myoclonic jerks.

Other antipsychotics associated with epileptiform activity are olanzapine (the second most common), phenothiazines, haloperidol, and risperidone, with quetiapine being closest to control groups. Haloperidol, ziprasidone, fluphenazine, pimozide, and risperidone are noted to exhibit relatively low risk.

Stimulant medication and drugs

The question of the safety of CNS stimulants in those with epilepsy is not uncommon as attention difficulties and epilepsy can be comorbid. If

the epilepsy is well controlled, increased seizures are generally not seen in patients on stimulants. However, in uncontrolled or refractory epilepsy, methylphenidate has been shown to increase seizures. Stimulants can increase the abundance of alpha and beta in the EEG and decrease the overall voltage. Stimulants, not surprisingly, increase the amount of time spent in N1 sleep and have been reported to decrease slow wave and REM sleep. Intoxication with stimulants at high doses can show an abnormal and encephalopathic EEG with diffuse slowing and epileptiform abnormalities.

Cocaine and amphetamines increase the amount of beta activity in the EEG. Cocaine is well known to lower the seizure threshold in people with epilepsy and in people with no prior history of seizures. Cocaine has been known to cause status epilepticus.

THE ROLE OF THE EEG IN DETERMINING ANTISEIZURE DRUG TREATMENT

The EEG plays a useful role in selecting an appropriate ASM. Although there may be sufficient information to make an informed decision on the basis of the clinical picture, this can be misleading. For example, in cases of tonic-clonic convulsions it is not necessarily obvious whether the seizures are primarily generalized or focal to bilateral tonic-clonic seizures. Likewise, in patients with apparent absence seizures, the clinical differentiation from focal impaired awareness seizures may be difficult. In both these instances the EEG offers assistance.

In individuals with absence seizures, one should select an agent that might be considered as an "anti-spike-wave" ASM, such as valproate. Topiramate and lamotrigine are also considerations. If the EEG picture and clinical evidence are diagnostic of absence epilepsy without concomitant GTC seizures or myoclonus, ethosuximide is an excellent choice. If the EEG reveals a temporal spike focus in a patient with apparent confusional states, a focal (e.g., eslicarbazepine acetate) or a broad-spectrum agent (e.g., levetiracetam, lamotrigine) could be used. If, on the other hand, the EEG is indeterminate (the EEG might be normal!), then selection of a broad-spectrum agent is indicated (e.g., levetiracetam, valproic acid, clobazam, lamotrigine, topiramate, or zonisamide). Older agents, such as phenytoin, valproate, or phenobarbital, have a higher side-effect profile and are usually not first-line choices. Some of the agents used to treat focal epilepsy, particularly carbamazepine, oxcarbazepine, eslicarbazepine, phenytoin, gabapentin, pregabalin and vigabatrin, may make generalized epilepsy worse, particularly absence seizures.

Newer ASMs include stiripentol approved for Dravet syndrome, fenfluramine for the treatment of Dravet syndrome and LGS, and cenobamate and brivaracetam for focal seizures.

Further reading

Abu-Khalil, B.W., 2019. Update on antiepileptic drugs 2019. Continuum (Minneap. Minn.). 25, 508–536.

Bauer, G., Bauer, R., 2011. EEG, drug effects and central nervous system poisoning. In: Schomer, D.L., Lopes da Silva, F.H. (Eds.), Niedermeyer's Electroencephalography: Basic Principles, Clinical Applications, and Related Fields, 6 ed. Lippincott Williams & Wilkins Health, Philadelphia, PA.

Blume, W.T., 2006. Drug effects on EEG. J. Clin. Neurophysiol 23, 306–311.

Eriksson, A.S., Knutsson, E., Nergardh, A., 2001. The effect of lamotrigine on epileptiform discharges in young patients with drug-resistant epilepsy. Epilepsia 42, 230–236.

French, J.A., Pedley, T.A., 2008. Clinical practice. Initial management of epilepsy. N. Engl. J. Med. 359, 166–176.

Gibbs, F.A., Gibbs, E.L., Lennox, W.G., 1937. Effect on the electroencephalogram of certain drugs which influence nervous activity. Arch. Intern. Med. 60, 154–166.

Goyal, N., Praharaj, S.K., Desarkar, P., et al., 2011. Electroencephalographic abnormalities in clozapine-treated patients: a cross-sectional study. Psychiatry Investig. 8, 372–376.

Grayson, L., Ampah, S., Hernando, K., et al., 2021. Longitudinal impact of cannabidiol on EEG measures in subjects with treatment-resistant epilepsy. Epilepsy Behav. 122, 108190.

Grill, M.F., Maganti, R.K., 2011. Neurotoxic effects associated with antibiotic use: management considerations. Br. J. Clin. Pharmacol. 72, 381–393.

Haider, J., Matthew, H., Oswald, J., 1971. Electroencephalographic changes in acute drug poisoning. Electroencephalogr. Clin. Neurophysiol. 30, 23–31.

Harvey, S.C., 1975. Hypnotics and sedatives. The barbiturates. In: Goodman, L.S., Gilman, A. (Eds.), The Pharmacological Basis of Therapeutics. Macmillan, New York, pp. 102–123.

Herkes, G.K., Lagerlund, T.D., Sharbrough, F.W., et al., 1993. Effects of antiepileptic drug treatment on the background frequency of EEGs in epileptic patients. J. Clin. Neurophysiol. 10, 210–216.

Huang, C.W.W., Brown, S., Pillay, N., et al., 2018. Electroencephalographic and electrocardiographic effect of intravenous lacosamide in refractory focal epilepsy. J. Clin. Neurophysiol. 35, 365–369.

Jackson, A., Seneviratne, U., 2019. EEG changes in patients on antipsychotic therapy: a systematic review. Epilepsy Behav. 95, 1–9.

Kochen, S., Giagante, B., Oddo, S., 2002. Spike-wave complexes and seizure exacerbation caused by carbamazepine. Eur. J. Neurol. 9, 41–47.

Marciani, M.G., Stanzione, P., Maschio, M., et al., 1997. EEG changes induced by vigabatrin monotherapy in focal epilepsy. Acta Neurol. Scand. 95, 115–120.

Marciani, M.G., Stanzione, P., Mattia, D., et al., 1998. Lamotrigine add-on therapy in focal epilepsy: electroencephalographic and neuropsychological evaluation. Clin. Neuropharmacol. 21, 41–47.

Szaflarski, J.P., 2004. Effects of zonisamide on the electroencephalogram of a patient with juvenile myoclonic epilepsy. Epilepsy Behav. 5, 1024–1026.

Veauthier, J., Haettig, H., Meencke, H.J., 2009. Impact of levetiracetam add-on therapy on different EEG occipital frequencies in epileptic patients. Seizure 18, 392–395.

Wise, A., Lemus, H.N., Fields, M., et al., Refractory Seizures Secondary to Vitamin B6 Deficiency in Parkinson Disease: The Role of Carbidopa-Levodopa. Case Rep Neurol. 2022 Jun 27;14(2):291–295.

Wanleenuwat, P., Suntharampillai, N., Iwanowski, P., 2020. Antibiotic-induced epileptic seizures: mechanisms of action and clinical considerations. Seizure 81, 167–174.

In status epilepticus each case must be individually analyzed. The treatment of epilepsia partialis continua will be far less aggressive than the treatment of convulsive status epilepticus. However, certain tenets remain the same. In every patient who has status epilepticus, the first step is heeding the basics and making sure that airway, breathing, and circulation are secure. If intravenous (IV) access has been achieved, then thiamine and glucose along with an abortive medication (for example, lorazepam 0.1 mg/kg) are given. If there is no IV access, intramuscular (IM) midazolam is an excellent alternative. An underlying cause, particularly those that are easily reversible (hypoglycemia) or life-threatening (meningitis or an epidural hematoma), is sought with physical examination, lab tests, imaging, and a lumbar puncture if needed.

After an initial dose of a benzodiazepine, all cases of status epilepticus should be followed by a loading dose (LD) of an appropriate IV antiseizure medication (ASM). The Established Status Epilepticus Treatment Trial (ESSET) randomized patients with convulsive status epilepticus refractory to IV benzodiazepines to an IV load of fosphenytoin (20 phenytoin equivalents [PE]/kg), valproic acid (40 mg/kg), or levetiracetam (60 mg/kg) in the emergency setting. This study found no significant difference in the clinical cessation of seizure activity as determined by clinically evident seizures and mental status assessments among the three agents. Therefore, any of the above ASMs may be reasonable choices depending on the clinical scenario. For adults with presumed focal epilepsy, fosphenytoin under cardiac monitoring is often considered a first-line agent. However, fosphenytoin should be avoided in individuals (usually children) who have a known myoclonic form of epilepsy. In this instance, valproate is a reasonable choice in children older than 2 years of age. Likewise, as a broad-spectrum agent, levetiracetam, may also be used for several seizure types, but perhaps avoided when there is a clinical history of psychiatric disease. If seizures do not break after an initial benzodiazepine and a load of an IV ASM, the next step for convulsive seizures is intubation and preparation for a continuous infusion. Addition of another ASM before intubation can be considered; however, if the patient has been seizing for more than 30 minutes, it is recommended to start continuous anesthetic infusion with boluses.

The goal of treatment of status epilepticus is eradication of both electrographic and clinical signs of seizures, as well as appropriate diagnosis and treatment of any underlying condition causing the status epilepticus. Any individual that clinically remits but who is not back to baseline must be connected to a continuous video-EEG (VEEG) as there is often no clinical difference between a postictal state and ongoing nonconvulsive status epilepticus (NCSE). While experts may argue on how deep the EEG suppression should be, all would agree that the infusion should suppress all electrographic seizures. For treatment of nonconvulsive seizures detected on EEG, the Treatment of Recurrent Electrographic

Nonconvulsive Seizures (TRENdS) trial showed noninferiority of loading IV lacosamide (400 mg) compared to fosphenytoin (20 PE/kg). Choice of other additional agents largely depends on the patient and comorbid conditions. For example, if the patient is acidotic, topiramate would be a poor choice as it can cause metabolic acidosis. IV LDs for ASMs as well as important adverse events are listed in Table Appendix 2.1.

Dosing guidelines for both intermittent bolus medication and continuous infusions for the treatment of status epilepticus are based on recent consensus guidelines from the Neurocritical Care Society and several recent reviews; however, randomized controlled data are lacking (Table Appendix 2.1). Initial anesthetic medications usually include midazolam and/or propofol. Ketamine is increasingly used as an adjunctive therapy. After anesthetics infusions are started, epileptologists will generally aim for a period of seizure freedom with or without burst suppression lasting at least 24 hours before gradually tapering the continuous infusion.

All cases of status epilepticus require a comprehensive workup for etiology, which may be diverse, including noncompliance with seizure medications in patients with epilepsy, acute brain pathology (including stroke, brain hemorrhage, traumatic brain injury and meningitis/encephalitis), metabolic derangements, autoimmune and paraneoplastic causes. For patients with new-onset refractory status epilepticus (NORSE) or autoimmune encephalitis, additional treatments including immune therapy with steroids, intravenous immune globulin, plasmapheresis, rituximab, and anakinra may be considered. Additionally, nonpharmacologic therapies such as the ketogenic diet and surgical therapy (resection of an epileptogenic lesion or vagal nerve stimulation) could be considered in select cases.

Table Appendix 2.1 Dosing in status epilepticus

Drug	Initial dosing	Administration rates and alternative dosing recommendations	Serious adverse effects	Considerations
Initial Treatment with Benzodiazepines				
Diazepam	LD: 0.25 mg/kg IV push up to 10 mg per dose, repeat every 5 min until seizures stop up to 3 doses or 30 mg MD: n/a	Up to 5 mg/min (IVP) Peds: 2–5 years, 0.5 mg/kg (PR); 6–11 years, 0.3 mg/kg (PR); older than 12 years, 0.2 mg/kg (PR)	Hypotension, respiratory depression	Rapid redistribution, longer half-life compared to other benzodiazepines, active metabolite, IV contains propylene glycol; may cause metabolic acidosis
Lorazepam	LD: 0.1 mg/kg IV up to 4 mg per dose, repeat every 5 min until seizures stop up to 3 doses or 12 mg MD: n/a	Up to 2 mg/min (IVP)	Hypotension, respiratory depression	Rapid redistribution, dilute 1:1 with saline, IV contains propylene glycol; may cause metabolic acidosis

Table Appendix 2.1 Dosing in status epilepticus—cont'd

Drug	Initial dosing	Administration rates and alternative dosing recommendations	Serious adverse effects	Considerations
Midazolam (also used as a continuous infusion)	LD: 0.2 mg/kg IV (max 20 mg), repeat 0.2–0.4 mg/kg IV boluses (max 40 mg per bolus) every 5 min until seizures stop, max total dose 2 mg/kg MD: 0.1–2.9 mg/kg/h, titrate to seizure suppression	0.2 mg/kg (up to 10 mg) IM (>40 kg); 5 mg IM (13–40 kg); 0.2 mg/kg (intranasal); 0.5 mg/kg (buccal), consider dose reduction in renal or hepatic impairment	Respiratory depression, hypotension	Active metabolite, renal elimination, rapid redistribution (short duration)
ASMs for Status Epilepticus				
Fosphenytoin	LD: 20 mg PE/kg IV (max 2000 mg), may give additional 5 mg/kg if still seizing MD: use phenytoin	Up to 150 mg PE/min; may give additional dose 10 min after loading infusion Peds: up to 3 mgPE/kg/min Reduce dose in renal or hepatic impairment	Hypotension, arrhythmias	Compatible in saline, dextrose, and lactated ringer solutions
Lacosamide	LD: 10 mg/kg IV (max 500 mg), may give additional 5 mg/kg (max 250 mg) if still seizing MD: 200–600 mg/day divided q6h–q12h	Over 5–10 min, max IV push dose of 400 mg at a rate of 80 mg/min No pediatric dosing established Reduce dose in severe renal impairment, max 300 mg per day	PR prolongation, atrial fibrillation, hypotension	Minimal drug interactions
Levetiracetam	60 mg/kg IV (max 4500 mg) Peds: 20–60 mg/kg IV	2–5 mg/kg/min, max IV push dose of 1500 mg at a rate of 500 mg/min Reduce dose in renal impairment		Minimal drug interactions, not hepatically metabolized, may cause behavioral disturbance
Phenobarbital	LD: 15 mg/kg IV (max dose 1500 mg), may give an additional 5–10 mg/kg if still seizing MD: 1–3 mg/kg/day given every day or divided q12h	50–100 mg/min IV, may give additional dose 10 min after loading infusion Reduce dose in renal or hepatic impairment	Hypotension, respiratory depression	IV contains propylene glycol; may cause metabolic acidosis, strong P450 inducer, dose adjustment of other ASMs might be necessary

(Continued)

Table Appendix 2.1 Dosing in status epilepticus—cont'd

Drug	Initial dosing	Administration rates and alternative dosing recommendations	Serious adverse effects	Considerations
Phenytoin	LD: 20 mg/kg IV, may give an additional 5–10 mg/kg MD: 200–600 mg/day divided q12h or q8h	Up to 50 mg/min IV Peds: up to 1 mg/kg/min Reduce dose in renal or hepatic impairment	Arrhythmias, hypotension, purple glove syndrome	Only compatible in saline, IV contains propylene glycol; may cause metabolic acidosis, generally avoid use with most CYP3A4 substrates. Coadministration with valproate displaces phenytoin from protein binding site and induces metabolism of valproate
Valproate sodium	LD: 40 mg/kg IV (max 4000 mg), may give an additional 20 mg/kg (max 2000 mg) if still seizing MD: 2000–6000 mg divided q8h–q6h	3–6 mg/kg/min, may give additional dose 10 min after loading infusion Peds (older than 2 years): 1.5–3 mg/kg/min Caution in hepatic impairment	Hyperammonemia, pancreatitis, thrombocytopenia, platelet dysfunction, hepatotoxicity	Phenytoin and valproate may displace each other from protein binding sites. Concurrent use with carbapenems (imipenem, meropenem, ertapenem) results in decreased level of valproate
Continuous Infusions for Status Epilepticus (midazolam dosing in the above section)				
Propofol	1–2 mg/kg IV bolus via infusion pump; max dose 200 mg, repeat q3–5 min until seizures stop; max total load of 10 mg/kg	Initial: 30 mcg/kg/min CI. Maintenance: 30–200 mcg/kg/min; titrate to seizure suppression. Use caution when administering high doses (>80 mcg/kg/min) for extended periods of time (i.e., >48 h) Peds: Use caution with doses >65 mcg/kg/min; contraindicated in young children	Hypotension, respiratory depression, cardiac failure, rhabdomyolysis, metabolic acidosis, renal failure, PRIS	Requires mechanical ventilation, must adjust daily caloric intake (1.1 kcal/mL)
Ketamine	1.5 mg/kg IV (push over 3–5 min); max 150 mg repeat until seizures stop; max LD 4.5 mg/kg	Initial 1.2 mg/kg/h; maintenance 0.3–7.5 mg/kg/h; titrate to seizure suppression Consider dose reduction in hepatic impairment	Metabolic acidosis, hypertension, increased cerebral blood flow, psychiatric emergence phenomenon, neurotoxicity	NMDA antagonist, caution use in patients with uncontrolled hypertension, may elevate ICP, renal failure, or hepatic failure

Table Appendix 2.1 Dosing in status epilepticus—cont'd

Drug	Initial dosing	Administration rates and alternative dosing recommendations	Serious adverse effects	Considerations
Pentobarbital	5 mg/kg IV at 50 mg/min; max dose 500 mg; repeat until seizures stop; max total load of 25 mg/kg	Initial 1 mg/kg/h; maintenance: 0.5–10 mg/kg/h CI; titrate to seizure suppression Consider dose reduction in hepatic impairment	Hypotension, respiratory depression, cardiac depression, paralytic ileus At high doses, complete loss of neurological function	Requires mechanical ventilation, IV contains propylene glycol; may cause metabolic acidosis Prolonged half-life (up to 50 h, dose dependent)

ASMs, Antiseizure medications; *CI*, continuous infusion; *h*, hour; *ICP*, intracranial pressure; *IM*, intramuscular; *IV*, intravenous; *IVP*, intravenous push; *LD*, loading dose; *MD*, maintenance dose; *min*, minute; *n/a*, not applicable; *NMDA*, N-methyl-ᴅ-aspartate; *PE*, phenytoin equivalents; *Peds*, pediatric; *PR*, rectal administration, *PRIS*, propofol-related infusion syndrome; *q6h (q8h, q12h)*, every 6 (8, 12) hours.

Further reading

Brophy, G.M., Bell, R., Claassen, J., et al., 2012. Guidelines for the evaluation and management of status epilepticus. Neurocrit. Care 17, 3–23.

Glauser, T., Shinnar, S., Gloss, D., et al., 2016. Evidence-based guideline: treatment of convulsive status epilepticus in children and adults: Report of the Guideline Committee of the American Epilepsy Society. Epilepsy Curr. 16, 48–61.

Hirsch, L.J., Gaspard, N., van Baalen, A., et al., 2018. Proposed consensus definitions for new-onset refractory status epilepticus (NORSE), febrile infection-related epilepsy syndrome (FIRES), and related conditions. Epilepsia 59, 739–744.

Husain, A.M., Lee, J.W., Kolls, B.J., et al., 2018. Randomized trial of lacosamide versus fosphenytoin for nonconvulsive seizures. Ann. Neurol. 83, 1174–1185.

Kapur, J., Elm, J., Chamberlain, J.M., et al., 2019. Randomized trial of three anticonvulsant medications for status epilepticus. N. Engl. J. Med. 381, 2103–2113.

Norse institute: https://www.norseinstitute.org/.

Trinka, E., Leitinger, M., 2022. Management of status epilepticus, refractory status epilepticus, and super-refractory status epilepticus. Continuum (Minneap Minn). 28, 559–602.

Young, G.B., Mantia, J., 2017. Continuous EEG monitoring in the intensive care unit. Handb. Clin. Neurol. 140, 107–116.

Active sleep. Seen in the neonatal EEG. Typically, the EEG is continuous, there are rapid eye movements (REMs), low muscle tone, and irregular respirations.

Activité moyenne. Means "average or medium" and refers to the normal full-term neonatal awake and active sleep background. This consists of continuous, low- to medium-voltage activity predominantly in the theta and delta range with overriding beta.

Alpha. Frequencies in the range of 8 to <13 Hz.

Alpha coma. Infrequently seen after a catastrophic brain injury such as anoxia. The patient is comatose, and the EEG shows alpha range activity in a widespread distribution, usually maximal in the frontal regions. There is no reactivity as seen with the PDR. Prognosis is poor.

Alpha variants. Variants of the PDR with harmonically related frequencies. Slow alpha variant is half the alpha frequency; fast alpha variant is twice the alpha frequency. May coexist with alpha or appear alone. Notched appearance of slow alpha variant gives a clue to its presence.

Amplitude. The voltage of the waveform. Measured in microvolts (μV).

A-P gradient. Anterior-posterior gradient. In a normal awake adult EEG there are faster frequencies that are lower in amplitude anteriorly and a well-formed PDR occipitally.

Asynchrony. The opposite of synchrony—that is, the independent or nonsimultaneous occurrence of EEG waves over the two hemispheres.

Attenuation. Reduction of EEG activity. An example is reduction or disappearance of the alpha following eye opening.

Background. The underlying activity of the brain. Focal slow waves, synchronous bifrontal slowing, epileptiform discharges, and seizures are said to interrupt the background.

Band. Refers to a frequency range. For example, alpha lies in the 8–13 Hz frequency band.

Beta. Rhythmic, usually low-voltage activity at 13–30 Hz. Usually maximal over the frontocentral regions. Increases in amplitude and becomes more widespread with certain drugs (e.g., benzodiazepines, barbiturates).

Bilateral synchrony. Refers to waveforms appearing simultaneously over both hemispheres. A focal discharge spreads rapidly from one area of the brain to another and is indistinguishable on surface electrodes from a generalized discharge.

Bipolar recording. Recording that compares the activity at two neighboring electrodes with one electrode in input 1 and the second electrode in input 2 of the amplifier. The phase reversal is the localization principle of bipolar recording.

Breach rhythm. Term referring to localized increased amplitude of background rhythms with increased fast activity that result from an underlying craniotomy or break in the calvarium (Breach: a broken or torn place. *Webster's World College Dictionary*, 4th ed.). Beta activity with admixed slower frequencies may appear quite sharp and should not be mistaken for epileptiform discharges.

Brief potentially ictal rhythmic discharges (BIRDs). Focal or generalized rhythmic activity >4 Hz (at least six waves at a regular rate) lasting ≥0.5 to <10 seconds, not consistent with a known normal pattern or

GLOSSARY

benign variant, not part of burst suppression or burst attenuation, and without definite clinical correlate.

Burst suppression. Episodic or paroxysmal potentials, slow or sharp, or a combination of both, followed by suppression of cerebral activity. EEG is suppressed >50% of the time.

Channel. Refers to the output of an amplifier that displays electrical information. The number of channels displayed by an EEG apparatus varies.

Common average reference recording. Referential montage in which the activity from the exploring electrode is compared with the averaged activity of the remaining electrodes on the scalp.

Common mode rejection. A signal that is the same in the two amplifier inputs is "rejected" and not displayed, as there is no potential difference.

Common mode signal. Any activity, either physiological or environmental, that is the same at the two inputs of an amplifier.

Complex. The pattern of two or more distinct wave forms. The best example is the spike-wave complex in which each discharge has the same temporal relationship of the spike to the following wave.

Delta. Frequencies that are in the >0 to <4 Hz frequency band.

Delta brush. A slow, moderate- to high-amplitude delta wave with superimposed lower-amplitude fast frequencies. Common in the neonatal EEG. Also sometimes seen in persons with NMDA limbic encephalitis (called extreme delta brush).

Depression. Refers to reduction of amplitude or voltage due to a disease process, focal or generalized. An example would be the depression of amplitude sometimes recorded over a subdural hematoma or hygroma.

Derivation. Recording from an electrode pair with the output displayed in one channel of the recording.

Differential amplifier. An amplifier whose output is proportional to the difference in voltage between the two input terminals.

Diffuse. Occurring generally over the two hemispheres, usually used to describe slowing. Contrast with focal slowing.

Discharge. Epileptiform waveform (e.g., a sharp wave or polyspike) lasting <0.5 seconds regardless of the number of phases or >0.5 seconds with no more than three phases.

Electrode impedance. Opposition to AC current flow between an electrode and its interface with the scalp. Measured between pairs of electrodes and measured in ohms (<5 K ohms is recommended, <100 ohms suggests a salt bridge). It is important that electrode impedances are generally equal and relatively low in order to ensure good, artifact-free recording.

Electrographic seizure. Recorded ictal activity with or without clinical accompaniment. May be focal with recruiting rhythms or generalized.

Encoches frontales. Frontal sharp waves in the neonatal period, which may occur in isolation or in brief runs. These are normal.

Epilepsia partialis continua (EPC). Ongoing focal clonic motor seizures without impairment of consciousness. Often does not have an electrographic correlate.

Epileptiform discharges. Refers to BIRDs, polyspikes, spikes, spike-wave complexes, sharp waves, LPDs and LRDA.

Equipotential. Term used to indicate equal potentials at different electrodes.

Exploring electrode. The designation of an electrode that records cerebral activity of interest.

Fast activity. Synonym for beta or gamma activity.

Focus. Refers to the location of maximal potential, usually electronegative.

Fourteen and six positive spikes (14/6). Electropositive spikes at 14 or 6 Hz, or a combination of both. Usually maximal in the posterior temporal derivations and best recorded with wide interelectrode distances (e.g., the crossed ear reference). Of doubtful clinical significance.

Frontally predominant GRDA. High-voltage bifrontal rhythmic waves, which are nonspecific but may be indicative of increased intracranial pressure, deep structural lesions, toxic metabolic states, or other encephalopathies. If this activity appears during sleep onset in the elderly, it is considered normal.

Half alpha variant. Normal variant seen in children after age 8. One-half of the frequency of the PDR. Notched appearance.

High-frequency filter (aka low-pass filter). Attenuates high frequencies (passes all the low frequencies, filters out high frequencies). Can be adjusted by a stepped control available on all EEG machines and digital reading stations.

Hyperventilation. Standard procedure during routine EEG recording. The subject is asked to over-breathe deeply at a faster than normal rate for a period of 3–5 minutes. Often activates latent abnormalities, especially the generalized spike-wave discharges seen in childhood absence epilepsy.

Hypnogogic hypersynchrony. Diffuse semirhythmic high voltage slow waves lasting for several seconds in drowsiness. Seen in children older than 6 months of age.

Hypnopompic hypersynchrony. Diffuse semirhythmic high-voltage slow waves lasting for several seconds upon arousal. Seen in children older than 6 months of age.

Hypsarrhythmia. Chaotic, very high-voltage discharges consisting of an admixture of generalized spikes, sharp waves, and slow waves, characteristic of infantile epileptic spasms syndrome. One may also see focal discharges, as well as intermittent suppression of cerebral activity.

Input I. Refers to the first of two inputs to an amplifier (Lead 1).

Input II. Refers to the second of two inputs to an amplifier (Lead 2).

Interelectrode distance. Distance between pairs of electrodes.

Isolated. Refers to a waveform (e.g., a spike or slow wave) occurring as an individual, nonrepetitive event.

Isopotentiality. Term used for lack of electrocortical potentials. Seen after severe cerebral damage secondary to cardiopulmonary arrest or during deep anesthesia. Sometimes referred to as "flat line."

K-complexes. High-voltage mono- or multiphasic paroxysmal slow potentials often found with sleep spindles. Prominent during N2 sleep. May be triggered during sleep by a loud sound (knock) with no clinical signs of arousal or transition out of sleep.

Lambda waves. Electropositive sharp potentials recorded in the occipital regions (like an evoked potential), generated when a subject is visually scanning the environment (often while reading).

Lead. Refers to an electrode and its connection to the EEG machine.

Low-frequency filter (aka high-pass filter). Attenuates low frequencies (passes all the high frequencies, filters out low frequencies low frequencies).

Monorhythmic occipital delta. Runs of high amplitude posterior delta. Seen in premature neonates.

Montage. Term used to indicate the arrangement of electrodes displaying the EEG activity.

Multifocal sharp transients. Sharp waves seen throughout the EEG in normal neonates.

Mu rhythm. Mu rhythm is a normal finding. It appears as sharply contoured rhythmic waves at 7–11 Hz, maximal over the central regions. May be unilateral or bilateral. Attenuates with movement of the opposite upper extremity (e.g., making a fist) or even thinking about moving the contralateral arm.

Nasopharyngeal electrode. Relatively thin, insulated wire with an exposed tip, introduced through the nose, coming to rest as the back of the nasopharynx adjacent to the sphenoid bone. Records activity from the inferior temporal or frontal lobe. Used less frequently today secondary to discomfort and artifact (e.g., respiratory, swallowing, pulse).

Noise. Small currents in an EEG channel related to the machine circuitry, not physiological potentials.

Notch filter. A circuit that filters out a narrow band of frequencies specifically removing the most common electrical artifact (e.g., a 60 Hz notch filter [50 Hz in UK]). Particularly important when recording in ICU settings, where a variety of electrical equipment is in use.

Organization. A well-organized adult waking EEG usually contains PDR in the occipital regions, beta activity in the frontocentral regions, and little else. If the PDR is disrupted by slower frequencies, the record might be said to be somewhat disorganized with intermittent generalized slowing. If there is no PDR along with a great deal of generalized delta range slowing, the record might be said to be disorganized and slow.

Paradoxical alpha. Alpha rhythm that appears after eye opening, seen in drowsy subjects (the opposite of what happens in alert subjects).

Periodic discharges (PDs). A repetitive waveform at regular intervals for at least 6 cycles with a relative fixed interdischarge interval (the period). Can be generalized (GPDs) as is often seen after cardiac arrest or lateralized (LPDs) as can be seen in an area of cerebral infarction or tumor. These discharges can be blunted delta, sharp waves, spikes, or polyspikes.

Phantom spike-wave. A normal variant characterized by low-voltage 5–6 Hz spike wave discharges.

Phase reversal. Localization principle of bipolar recording. The electrical phenomena of interest (e.g., a sharp wave or spike) point toward each other in adjacent channels.

Photic driving. Response to intermittent photic stimulation recorded in the occipital regions. The evoked waves are time-locked to the flash rate. If there is a 1:1 response, it is termed *the fundamental*. If the response is twice the flash frequency, it is termed *a harmonic response*, and if half the frequency it is termed *the subharmonic*. All are normal.

Photomyoclonic response. Response to intermittent photic stimulation consisting of repetitive muscle action potentials, maximal in the frontal derivations, linked to the flash frequency. A normal response that ceases when the flash train stops.

Photoparoxysmal response. Generalized, synchronous epileptiform activity consisting of spike and polyspike wave complexes, maximal in the frontal regions, evoked by intermittent photic stimulation. When recorded, the technician must stop the flash stimulus immediately to avoid the possibility of precipitating a generalized seizure. The response can outlast cessation of the flash train by 1–2 seconds. The response is not always convulsive in nature.

Photosensitivity. General term used both for seizures triggered by flashing light and for epileptiform discharges evoked by photic stimulation in the EEG lab (the photoparoxysmal response). With lesser degrees of photosensitivity, occipital spikes or generalized spikes or sharp waves are time-locked to the flash frequency. People with certain types of epilepsy (like juvenile myoclonic epilepsy or progressive myoclonic epilepsy) are often photosensitive.

Positive occipital sharp transients of sleep (POSTs). Electropositive sharp potentials (in a referential recording), maximal in the occipital derivations. May be quite prominent. Often noted during N2 sleep. May occur in rhythmic runs.

Posterior dominant rhythm (PDR). Consists of alpha frequency (8.5 to <13 Hz in a normal adult) in the posterior regions of the head. The PDR attenuates with eye opening and is best seen when the person is in the relaxed, waking state with eyes closed.

Posterior slow waves of youth. Occur commonly between 2 and 21 years of age. In the delta range, consisting of 3–6 fused alpha waves. Attenuates with eye opening like the PDR.

Postmenstrual age (PMA). PMA is the sum of the gestational age (the number of weeks since the last menstrual cycle) and the legal age (age since time of birth).

Psychogenic nonepileptic seizures (PNES). A seizure mimic thought to be a conversion or somatiform disorder.

Quiet sleep. In the newborn. Respirations are regular and the EEG can show a tracé discontinu, tracé alternant, or continuous pattern.

Reactivity. Alteration of EEG activity by external sensory stimulation. In a comatose patient, this is a favorable sign.

Reference recording. Electrodes in input 1 and 2 are not immediately adjacent on the scalp. In referential recording the activity from an exploring electrode (input 1) is compared with the reference, which is out of the field of interest, e.g., the ear (A1/A2) or vertex (Cz) (input 2). In referential recording, the localization principle is amplitude.

REM sleep. Rapid eye movement sleep. Stage of sleep characterized by rapid eye movements, loss of muscle tone, and yes, dreams.

Rhythmic delta activity (RDA). Rhythmic delta activity lasting for at least six cycles with no interval between each delta wave. Can be lateralized (LRDA) or generalized (GRDA). LRDA is associated with higher seizure rates.

Rhythmic midtemporal theta (RMTD). Normal variant. Rhythmic 4–7 Hz waves in the temporal regions, recorded during drowsiness. May be notched in appearance.

Sensitivity. Ratio of input voltage to output recorded in a channel of the EEG recording.

Sharp-slow complex. Epileptiform pattern consisting of a sharp wave followed by a slow wave, usually in the delta frequency band. A typical example is the generalized sharp-slow complex at 2 Hz, typical of Lennox–Gastaut syndrome.

Sharp wave. Paroxysmal sharp potential with duration of 70–200 ms. These are longer in duration than spikes but with very similar significance.

Sleep. Five stages categorized as N1 (attenuation of the PDR, appearance of vertex waves and POSTs), N2 (sleep spindles and K-complexes), N3 (slow wave), and REM (low muscle tone and dreaming). The N stands for non-REM. Each stage is progressively deeper sleep with slower brain waves.

Sleep spindles. Rhythmic, sometimes spindle-shaped activity at 12 to 14 Hz (±2), indicative of N2 sleep. Usually maximal over the central region. These waves are mediated by cells in the nucleus reticularis of the thalamus.

Slowing. Brain waves that oscillate at a slower frequency than what would be expected for a particular region. Can be focal or generalized. Can be monomorphic or polymorphic.

Small sharp spikes (SSS). (aka benign epileptiform transients of sleep). Low-amplitude, rapid spikes. They appear in both hemispheres usually asynchronously, most often in the temporal derivations, and become evident during drowsiness and light sleep. Normal variant.

Sphenoidal electrodes. Insulated electrode wires with an exposed tip, introduced through the mandibular notch via a hollow needle. After the needle comes to rest near the foramen ovale, the needle is withdrawn. Records activity from the anterior tip of the temporal lobe.

Spike. Paroxysmal potential with duration of 20–70 ms. Typically sticks out and disrupts the background, has a pointy shape with an asymmetric rise and fall; followed by a slow wave.

Spike-wave complex. Spike followed by time-locked, high-voltage slow wave. Various frequency bands. Synchronous, rhythmic 3 Hz spike-wave runs are typical of absence seizures. Synchronous 4–5 Hz spike-wave runs are seen in people with generalized tonic-clonic seizures alone (GTCA). Irregular rapid spike-wave discharges are typical of juvenile myoclonic epilepsy (JME).

Spread. Activity spreading out from its site of origin (e.g., PDR that is represented anterior to the occipital regions).

Subclinical rhythmic electroencephalographic discharges of adults (SREDA). A normal variant. Can be mistaken for focal electrographic seizure activity.

Temporal sawtooth. Sharply contoured rhythmic theta in the temporal electrodes. Seen between 26 and 32 weeks PMA.

Theta. Waves in the 4 to <8 Hz frequency band. May be a normal finding or may indicate pathology. Some theta is acceptable in the normal waking adult EEG.

Tracé alternant. Normal pattern found in newborns during quiet sleep characterized by bursts of continuous activity alternating with periods of lower voltage. In tracé alternant, the interburst interval is shorter than in tracé discontinu and slightly higher in amplitude.

Tracé discontinu. The normal discontinuous tracing encountered in healthy preterm babies, which consists of bursts of high-voltage activity interrupted by low-voltage interburst periods.

Triphasic waves. Diffuse paroxysmal potentials associated with hepatic encephalopathy or other metabolic encephalopathies but can occur in a wide range of circumstances. Quite sharp in configuration with three phases, synchronous, maximal bifrontally. Can have an anterior to posterior lag with the first deflection happening slightly sooner anteriorly than posteriorly.

Vertex sharp waves. Recorded during N1 and N2 sleep. May be high voltage, isolated, or repetitive and can be as sharp as spikes. Usually maximal in the central regions (C3, C4, Cz).

Wicket spikes. Sharply contoured rhythmic frequencies varying from 7 to 11 Hz, maximal in the midtemporal derivations, occurring in brief runs. Normal variant.

Index

Page numbers followed by "*f*" indicate figures,
"*t*"indicate tables.

Epilepsy of infancy with migrating focal seizures (EIMFS), 138t–143t
Epilepsy with eyelid myoclonia (EEM), 138t–143t
Epileptic encephalopathy with spike-wave activation in sleep (EE-SWAS), 138t–143t
Epileptic spasm, 128t–129t
Epileptiform, 202
Epileptiform activity, 208, 210
Epileptiform burst suppression, 195f
Epileptiform discharges, 100–105, 149, 171
  centrotemporal, 106, 107f
  focal, location and significance of, 105–106
  frontal and frontopolar, 106, 108f
  interictal, in EEG report, 203t–205t
  interictal paroxysmal waveforms in, 100
  midline, 106
  occipital, 105
  occipital spikes in, 101f
  sharp wave in, 100
  spike, spike-wave complex and polyspikes in, 100, 101f, 102f, 103f
  temporal, 105
  temporal sharp wave in, 104f
Epileptiform potentials, 171
EPSPs. See Excitatory postsynaptic potentials (EPSPs)
Ethanol, 209
Ethosuximide, 151, 208, 210–211
Events, in EEG report, 203t–205t
Evolution, 114
Excessive beta activity, 44f
Excessive diffuse delta, 45
"Excessive" slowing, in theta range, 80
Excitatory postsynaptic potentials (EPSPs), 1, 7, 106

Exploring electrode, 11–12
Eye blink artifact, 24f, 109
  with prosthetic eye, 25f
Eyelid flutter, artifact with, 26f
Eyelid myoclonia seizures, 128t–129t

F
F3/F4 electrodes, 4t, 5–6
F7/F8 electrodes, 4t, 6–7
False lateralization, 106
Familial focal epilepsy with variable foci, 138t–143t
Fast activity, 95. See also Beta activity
Fast alpha variant, 53–58, 57f
Fast Fourier series transform (FFT) spectrogram, 190, 191f, 192f, 193f, 194f, 195f, 196f, 197f, 198f–199f
Febrile infection-related epilepsy syndrome (FIRES), 138t–143t
Febrile seizures (FS), 138t–143t
  in Dravet syndrome, 148
Febrile seizures plus (FS+), 138t–143t
FFT. See Fast Fourier series transform (FFT) spectrogram
Filter, notch, 18
Focal attenuation, 95–100, 97f
  focal increased fast activity in, 95–100, 98f
Focal delta activity, 43–45
Focal delta waves, 95
Focal epileptic seizures, 127
Focal increased fast activity, 95–100, 98f
Focal polymorphic delta activity, 45
Focal rhythmic delta activity, 45
Focal seizures, 128t–129t
  in focal slowing, 95

Focal slowing, 95, 96f
  in dementia, 171
Focal status epilepticus, 182, 184f
Focus, 11
Formed visual hallucinations, 105
Fosphenytoin, 213, 214t–217t
14 and 6 positive spikes, 64, 67f
Fpl/Fp2 electrodes, 4t, 5–6
Frontal epileptiform discharges, 106, 108f
Frontal lobe epilepsy, 159t
Frontally predominant generalized rhythmic delta activity, 109, 110f
Frontal sharp waves, 73–77, 78f, 90t–91t
Frontal spike, 108f
Frontal wave, 108f
Frontocentral head regions, 43
Frontopolar epileptiform discharges, 106, 108f
Fz, 4–5, 4t

G
Gabapentin, 210–211
Gelastic seizures, with hypothalamic hamartoma, 138t–143t
General anesthesia, 208
Generalized epileptic seizures, 127
Generalized paroxysmal fast activity (GPFA), 114, 122f
Generalized periodic discharges (GPDs), 109, 112f
  with triphasic morphology, 177, 178f
Generalized periodic discharges with admixed rhythmic activity (GPD+R), 117f
Generalized periodic discharges with superimposed fast activity (GPD+F), 116f